An Atlas of Surgical Anatomy

T0074651

An Atlas of
Surgical Anatomy

Surgical commentary by

Alain C Masquelet, MD

Illustrations by Léon Dorn

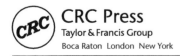

CRC Press
Taylor & Francis Group
Boca Raton London New York

CRC Press is an imprint of the
Taylor & Francis Group, an **informa** business

CRC Press
Taylor & Francis Group
6000 Broken Sound Parkway NW, Suite 300
Boca Raton, FL 33487-2742

First issued in paperback 2019

© 2005 by Taylor & Francis Group, LLC
CRC Press is an imprint of Taylor & Francis Group, an Informa business

No claim to original U.S. Government works

ISBN-13: 978-1-84184-405-3 (hbk)
ISBN-13: 978-0-367-39239-0 (pbk)

A CIP record for this book is available from the British Library.

Library of Congress Cataloging-in-Publication Data
Data avilable on application

Typeset by Scribe Design, Ashford, Kent

**Visit the Taylor & Francis Web site at
http://www.taylorandfrancis.com**

**and the CRC Press Web site at
http://www.crcpress.com**

Contents

Contents

Preface

Léon Dorn is one of the most famous medical illustrators in the world. Even today, at 80 years of age, he continues to pursue his work with the same enthusiasm. His work coincides with his great passion: the representation of the human body. Anatomy holds no secrets for him. He has spent countless hours in operating theatres, dissecting rooms and with himself; when Léon Dorn is drawing hands, he is drawing his own hands ...

Until recently, medical illustration was an undervalued job. The illustrators were basically artists, attracted to the human body. Many of them were self-trained people. Most of the time they were not well considered and some publishers even refused to mention their names in books.

Today, medical illustration has gained its 'letters patent of nobility'. Léon Dorn has witnessed the emergence, the development and the now well recognised state of the medical illustration.

Dorn is specially involved in the illustration of surgical techniques, which is probably the most difficult part of the art of medical illustration since the illustrator must attend surgical operations to understand what exactly is being done and then distil a long procedure into a few drawings. Usually, no more than five to seven drawings are needed to illustrate a surgical technique. The skill and possibly the genius of the artist lies in their ability to condense multiple operating stages into a limited number of drawings.

From a didactic point of view, it reveals the superiority of drawings over film. A film (movie or video sequence) delivers a linear succession of snap shots whereas a single drawing illustrates an entire sequence of a technical procedure.

For learning a technique, human understanding proceeds more by intuitive discerning of whole stages rather than separate elementary actions. This is the reason why the medical illustration based on drawings is superior to one based on videos. In spite of the recent advances in techniques of communi-cation, the illustrated book will always be valid for the learning process.

I would like just to comment upon Léon Dorn's manner of working. Some illustrators work at home, trying to restore a surgical technique from a draft prepared by the surgeon. Dorn's method is quite different. For him, the illustrator is like a reporter, an eye witness and a field worker; he has to perceive the intensity of an acute stage to express it through the drawing. This book is an attempt to communi-cate this particular state of mind. With Léon Dorn we have selected over 300 drawings from among a collection of several thousands.

These selected drawings do not constitute a treatise of surgical techniques. Their function is to highlight one of the main stages of the illustrator's work, which is the 'almost finished rough sketch'. For that reason the drawings are still outlines in lead pencil, in black and white. We have included a few definitive drawings in colour to show the contrast between what is actually published and what is the most important stage of the artist's work. Thus we present isolated drawings or several associated drawings, taken from different surgical fields, which do not constitute the complete description of a surgical technique.

The drawings are succinctly explained, just for understanding what they show. Where they are present, we have kept the legends written by the artist as an aid for the definitive drawing. On the other hand, we have not added new legends that could impede the serene contemplation of the drawings. What is important for the readers is to open their eyes for pleasure; the secret is not in the text but in the illustrations. Léon Dorn has rejuvenated the tradition of the medical illustrators who were initially artists admiring the human body, such as Calcar, the pupil of Le Titian, who immortalised the dissections of Vesalius, or Jacob, the pupil of David, who drew the anatomical preparations of Bourgery.

AC Masquelet

Léon Dorn
A biographical note

Léon Dorn was born in Paris in 1920. He lived in Israel from 1932 to 1965, where he worked in a kibbutz. This long stay in Israel was interrupted for two years (1953–1954) during which he studied at the Academy of Arts in Florence (Italy). In 1961, he was named general secretary of the Organisation of Painters and Sculptors of Kibboutzim.

He began to work as a medical illustrator when he came back to France in 1965. He was mostly commissioned by Masson Publishers and, in 1989, was invited by Professor Tubiana to illustrate surgical books for Martin Dunitz. His illustrations for *An Atlas of Flaps in Limb Reconstruction* (published by Martin Dunitz) won the Royal Society of Medicine Atlas award in 1995.

Léon Dorn is a pioneer of modern medical illustration in France. He actively participated in the efforts of the European Association of Medical and Scientific Illustrators to promote special schools devoted to medical illustration. A department was opened at the Ecole Estienne of Paris in 1992.

Léon Dorn
Notes on method

What is the method of Léon Dorn? Another form of this fascinating question could be: How is the genesis of a definitive drawing?

The secret of Léon Dorn is based on two principles:

1. An excellent knowledge of anatomy. As Léon Dorn has worked with many surgeons from different specialties, he has indepth knowledge of the anatomy of the human body. Moreover, he has contributed to several books on anatomy. It can be said that during his entire professional life Dorn has continued to compare anatomy as described and taught in books with real-life anatomy as encountered in operating rooms and theatres.

2. The second principle issues from the first. Léon Dorn draws 'live'. In his professional life he is permanently on the move to attend surgical operations and dissections. The vast majority of his illustrations have not been drawn from photographs or rough sketches made by surgeons but from what he has seen and observed.

The realisation of a definitive drawing as it will be published in a book has three important stages. It has been difficult to retrieve all the stages for one drawing from Dorn's archives. He has lost many drawings, and the first stage of a drawing is generally destroyed.

We have only one example of a complete series.

a) The first drawing is done in the operating room or in a theatre of anatomy. It can be called a sketch, but it is a very precise sketch. All the proportions are good, and all the structures are set in place: the nerves are coloured yellow, veins blue and arteries red. Some legends are added to remember exactly what has been drawn.

b) The second stage is drawn 'at home'. It is the intermediate stage between the sketch and the definitive drawing. It can be called the 'rough drawing'. Details are precisely drawn, for example the representation of the arteries and the thickness of the subcutaneous tissue. In this stage, primarily the shadows are applied to increase the impression of volume for the muscles and the perspective for the deep structures. The rough drawing is given to the surgeon who can then modify any detail on a tracing paper firmly attached to the drawing.

c) The definitive drawing is made once the rough drawing has been corrected. The structures are coloured or underlined in black ink and with paint.

The destiny of each stage is quite different:

- The sketches are generally destroyed or lost.
- The definitive drawing is given to the publisher and becomes their property.
- The intermediate stage – the rough drawing – which is, in fact, the most beautiful stage because it is the most realistic, remains the property of Léon Dorn.

Léon Dorn: notes on method

First stage

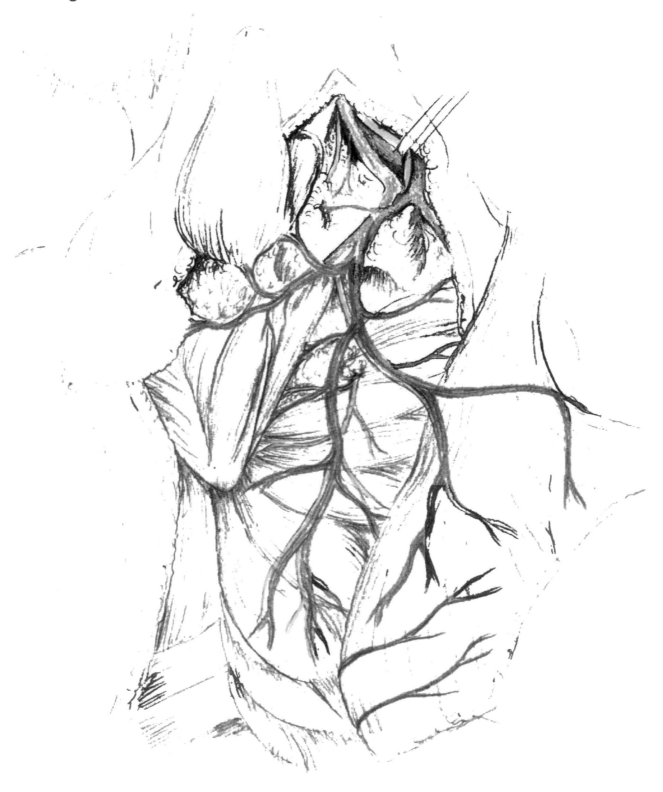

Second stage

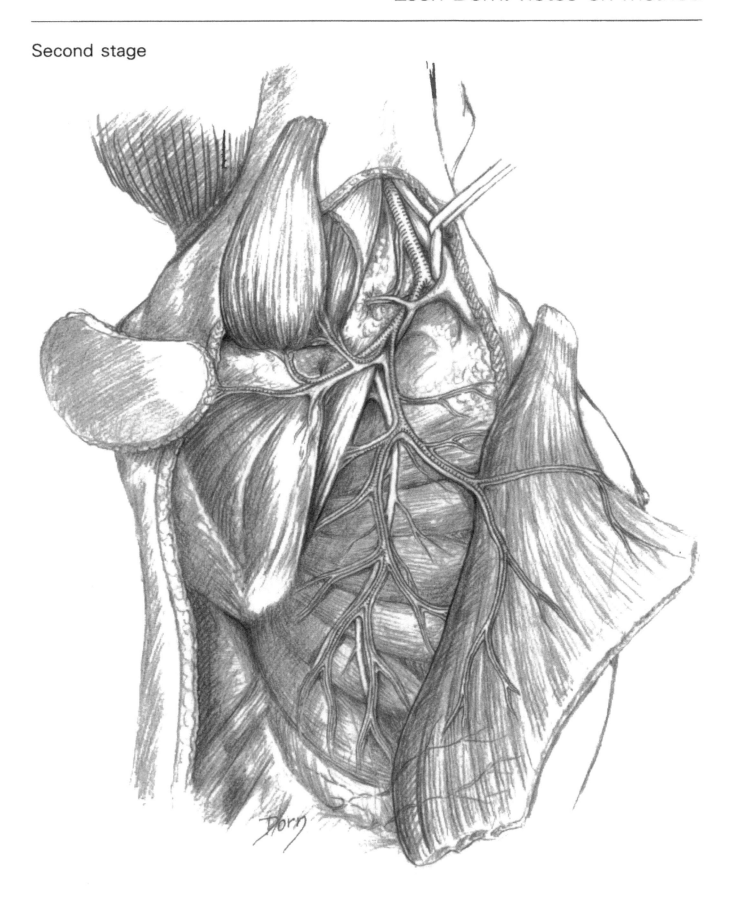

Third stage

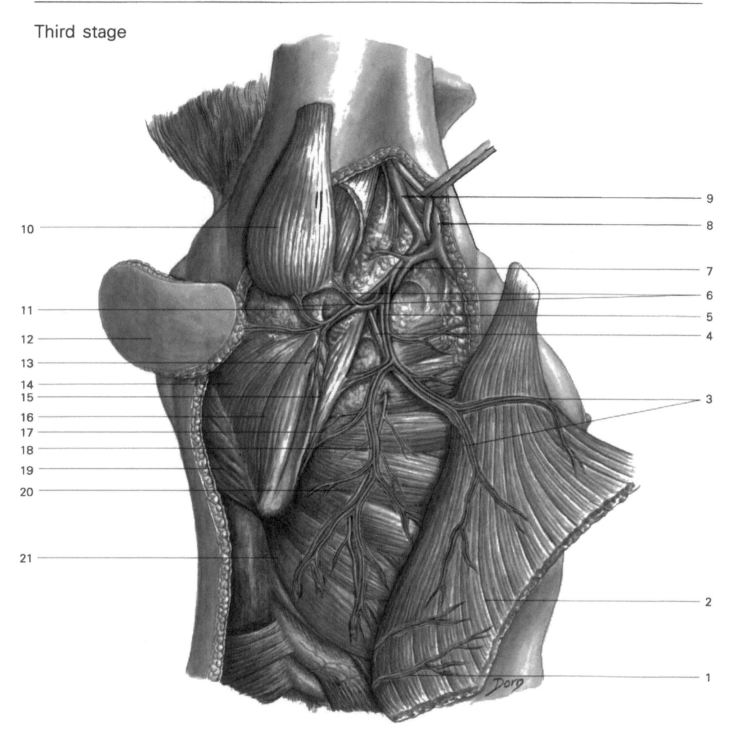

D

1 intramuscular pedicle issuing from
  intercostal arteries
2 latissimus dorsi muscle
3 intramuscular divisions of vascular
  pedicle supplying latissimus dorsi
4 nerve to latissimus dorsi
5 thoracodorsal pedicle
6 pedicles to teres major muscle

7 subscapular artery
8 axillary vein
9 axillary artery
10 teres major muscle
11 circumflex scapular artery and vein
12 scapular flap
13 vascular pedicle supplying rim of
   the scapula
14 infraspinatus muscle

15 subscapular muscle
16 teres minor muscle
17 bony angular branch to scapula
   (anastomoses with vascular
   pedicle supplying rim of scapula)
18 thoracic vessels
19 trapezius and rhomboid muscles
20 long thoracic nerve
21 serratus anterior muscle

1

Reconstructive surgery

During the past 30 years, reconstructive surgery has undergone incredible development. One of the main factors is microsurgical techniques which have permitted transfer of all kinds of tissue. There has been a renewed interest in anatomy, especially for the description of nutritive sources and vascular pedicles.

Recent advances in immunosuppressive treatment have allowed allotransplantation of functional organs, such as the hand.

An Atlas of Flaps of the Musculoskeletal System is the latest book illustrated by Léon Dorn. All the drawings are based on anatomical dissections and every detail is authentic.

Reconstructive surgery

Anatomy: the tree of flaps

The tree of flaps for the upper limb

Numerous flaps have been described.

The upper extremity is the source of fasciocutaneous flaps which can be used either as pedicled island flaps or as free revascularised flaps. The main vascular axis (the axillary artery or brachial artery) is considered as the trunk of the tree. Secondary arteries (such as the radial or ulnar artery) are the divisions of the trunk. The vascular pedicles of the flaps are formed from small branches and the flaps are the leaves.

1 latissimus dorsi flap
2 serratus anterior flap
3 scapular flaps
4 lateral arm flap
5 posterior intraosseous flap
6 radial forearm flap
7 distal ulnar flap
8 ulnar forearm flap

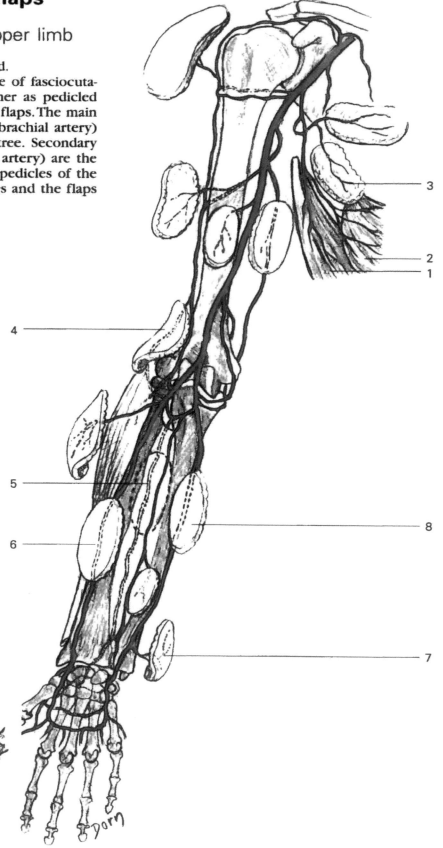

Flaps from the lower limb

Flap from the lateral head of the gastrocnemius

A The muscle is exposed with all the surrounding structures.

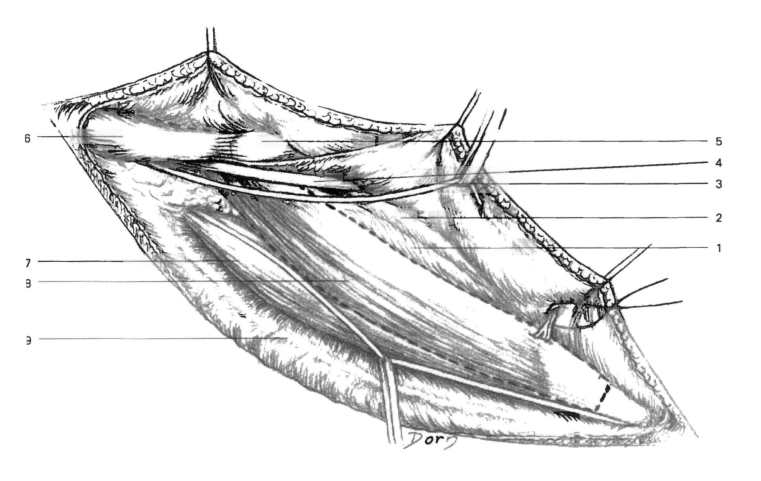

A

1 soleus
2 fibula
3 lateral sural cutaneous nerve
4 common peroneal nerve
5 head of fibula
6 biceps femoris
7 gastrocnemius (medial head)
8 gastrocnemius (lateral head)
9 lesser saphenous vein

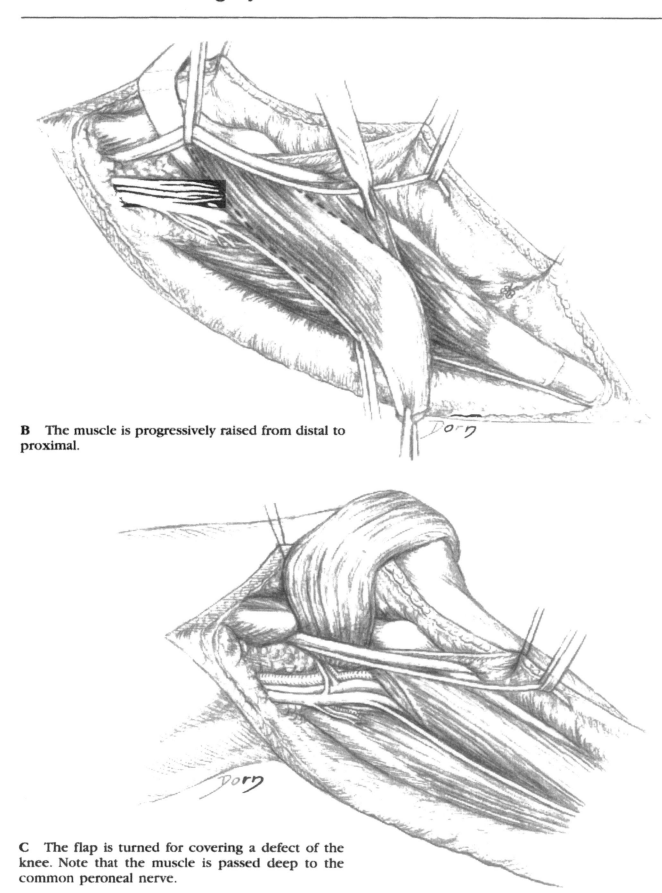

B The muscle is progressively raised from distal to proximal.

C The flap is turned for covering a defect of the knee. Note that the muscle is passed deep to the common peroneal nerve.

Soleus muscle flaps

This flap is suitable for covering a defect of the middle third of the leg.

A The muscle is exposed on the medial aspect of the leg. Two planes of dissection are developed: (i) between the soleus and the medial head of the gastrocnemius and (ii) between the soleus and the deep posterior compartment of the leg.

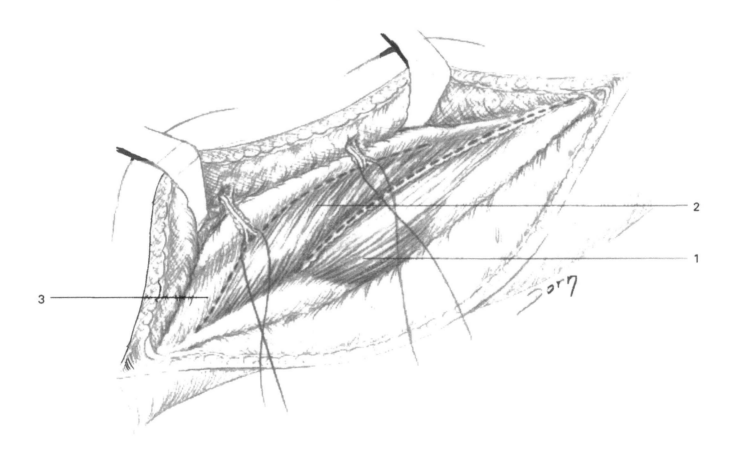

1 gastrocnemius (medial head)
2 soleus
3 deep posterior compartment

B, C   The distal portion of the soleus is isolated
and separated from Achilles' tendon.

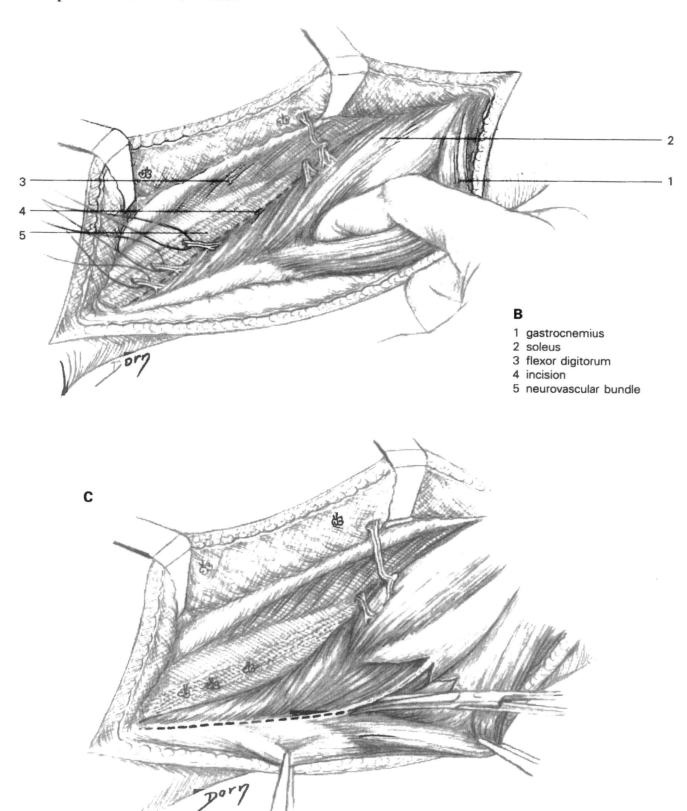

B

1 gastrocnemius
2 soleus
3 flexor digitorum
4 incision
5 neurovascular bundle

D The distal extremity of the muscle has been freed and the flap is raised from distal to proximal.

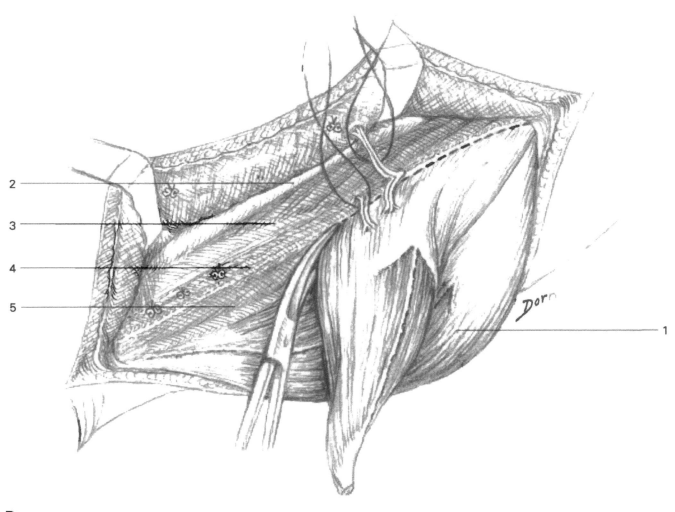

D

1 gastrocnemius
2 tibia
3 flexor digitorum longus
4 nerve and vessels
5 flexor hallucis longus

Reconstructive surgery

Sural skin flap

The sural skin flap is a neurocutaneous flap which is raised on the posterior aspect of the calf.

A The skin paddle is isolated on an adipofascial pedicle which contains a vein, superficial nerve and arterial network.

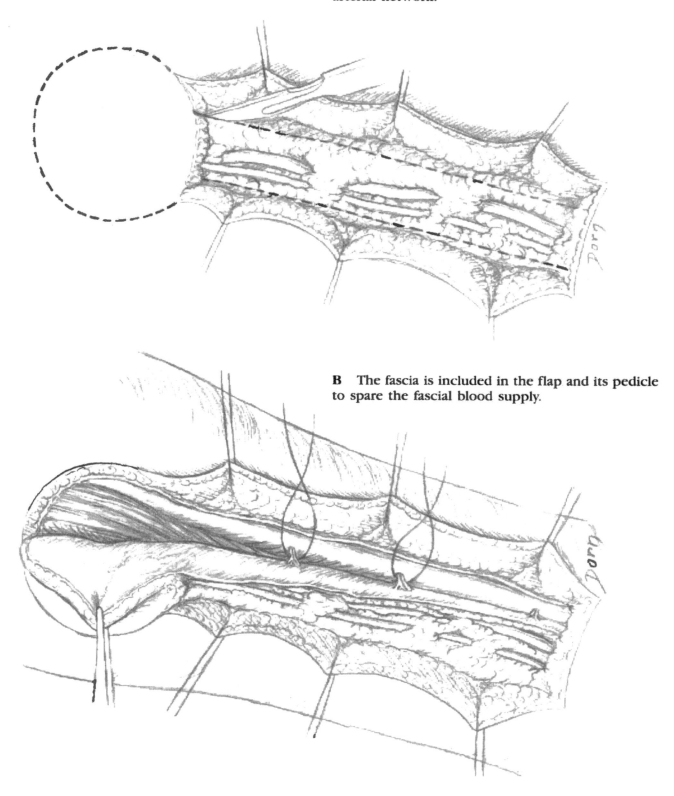

B The fascia is included in the flap and its pedicle to spare the fascial blood supply.

C   This flap is indicated for covering a defect over the posterior heel. It is supplied by a perforating vessel issued from the peroneal artery.

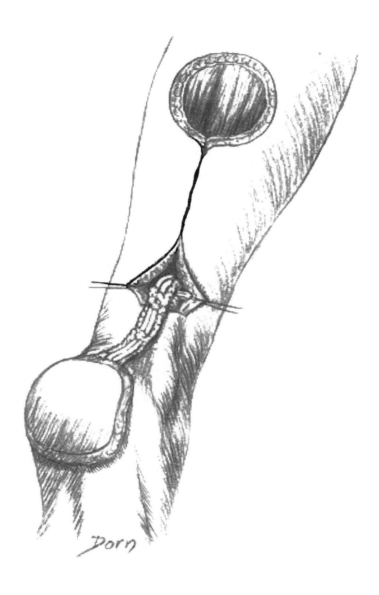

Vascularised bone transfers

Vascularised bone transfers have dramatically improved the treatment of bone defects. Healing occurs quickly avoiding the state of 'creeping substitution' specific to the revascularisation of conventional bone grafts.

Vascularised osteoperiosteal flap from the femur

This transfer is chiefly indicated in craniofacial surgery. It can also be used as a pedicled island flap to promote bone healing in a recalcitrant non-union of the femur.

The flap is detached from the medial aspect of the distal metaphysis of the femur. It is supplied by the descending genicular artery that issues from the lower femoral artery.

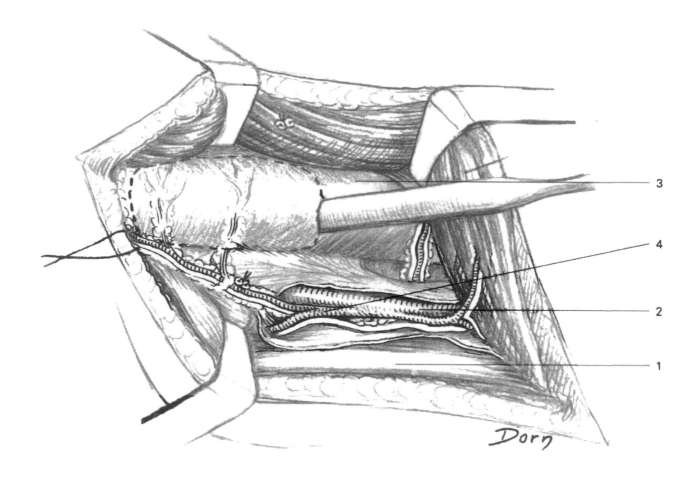

1 adductor magnus tendon
2 lower femoral artery
3 femur
4 descending genicular artery

Vascularised fibula transfer

The vascularised fibula is now of much interest in reconstructive surgery of long bone defects.

A   The fibula has been isolated with the peroneal vessels remaining protected by a portion of the tibialis posterior or the flexor hallucis longus muscles. The transfer is severed at both extremities, sparing a cuff of periosteum.

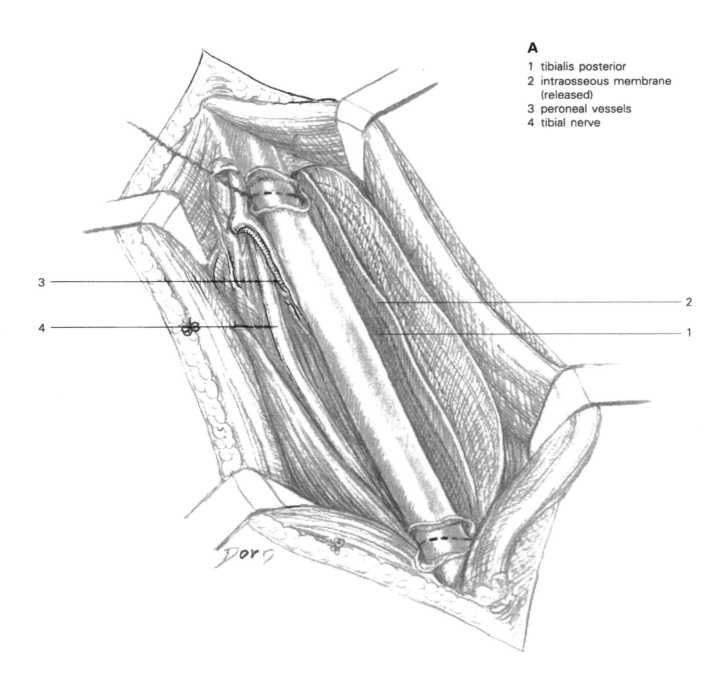

A
1 tibialis posterior
2 intraosseous membrane (released)
3 peroneal vessels
4 tibial nerve

B A portion of tibialis posterior muscle remains attached to the fibula to protect the peroneal vessels which supply the bone.

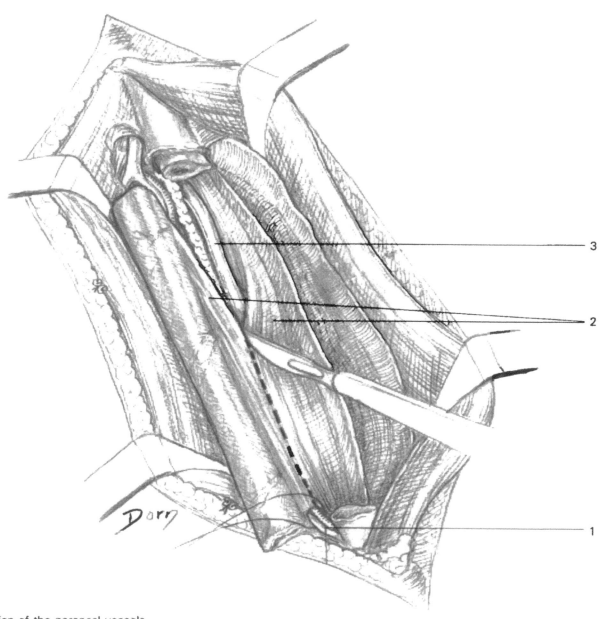

B

1 distal ligation of the peroneal vessels
2 tibialis posterior (split)
3 tibial nerve

C The transfer is completely isolated on its pedicle.

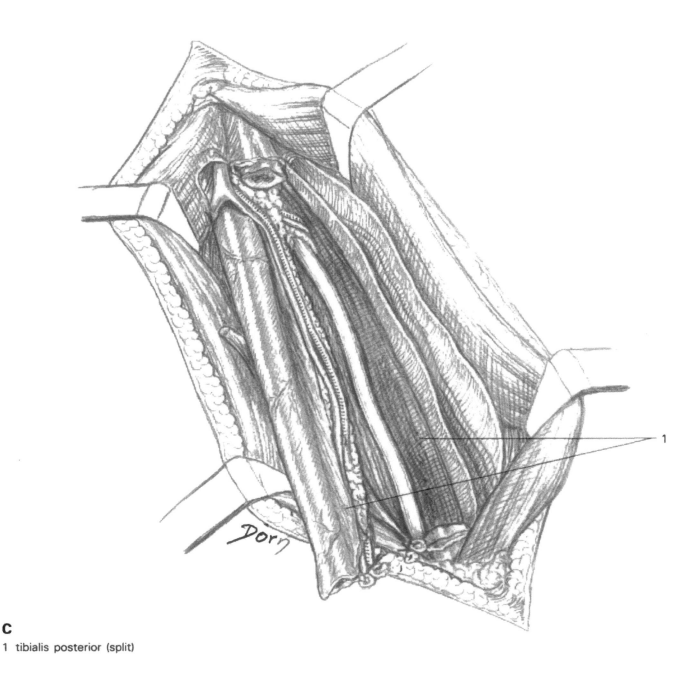

C

1 tibialis posterior (split)

Flaps from the upper limb

Lateral brachial flap

The lateral brachial flap is raised on the lateral aspect of the arm and is available as a pedicled flap or a free flap. It can be combined with a piece of bone from the humerus.

A Incision – the blood supply comes from the posterior branch of the brachial artery.

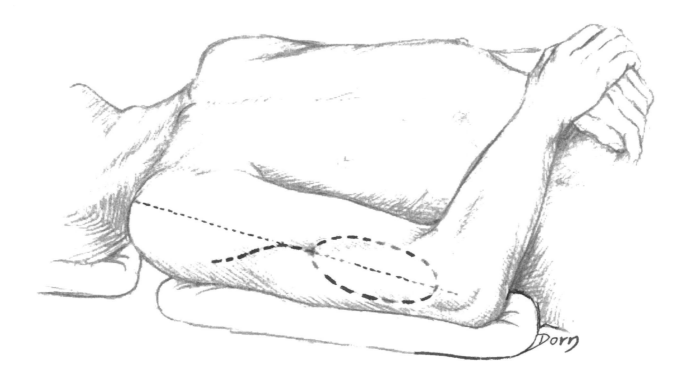

B The vessels are seen within the septum inserted on the humeral shaft.

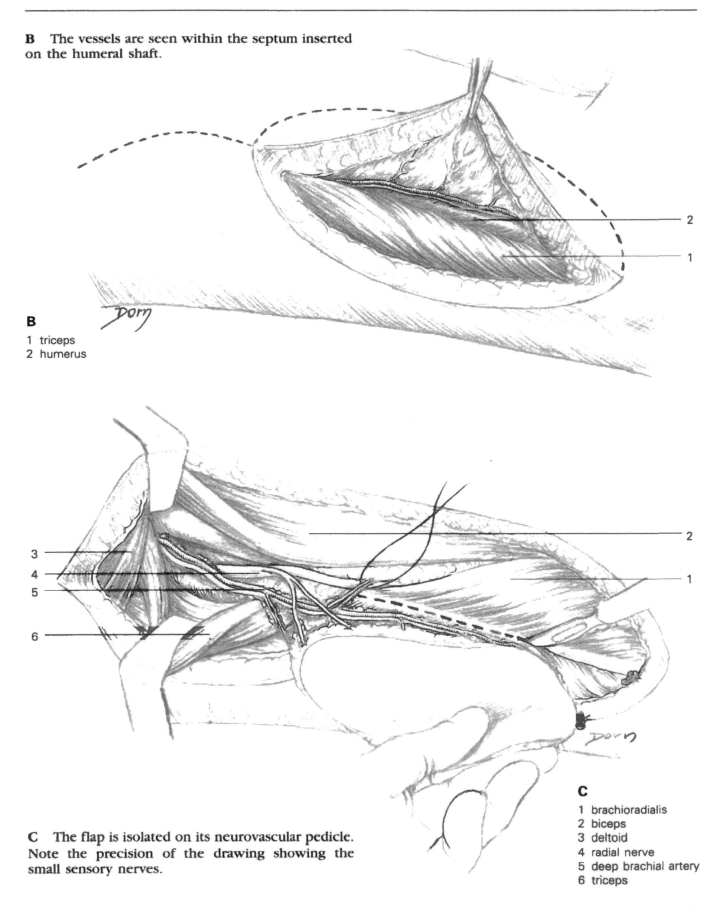

B

1 triceps
2 humerus

C The flap is isolated on its neurovascular pedicle. Note the precision of the drawing showing the small sensory nerves.

C

1 brachioradialis
2 biceps
3 deltoid
4 radial nerve
5 deep brachial artery
6 triceps

Reconstructive surgery

Forearm radial flap

This flap was the origin of a true revolution in 1980. Described by Chinese authors it is supplied by the radial artery and started the era of distally based pedicled island flaps, with retrograde blood flow, which were initially considered difficult to achieve.

A, B The flap is raised progressively on its vascular axis which is maintained in continuity during the first step of the dissection.

A
1 palmaris longus
2 flexor carpi radialis
3 radial artery
4 brachioradialis

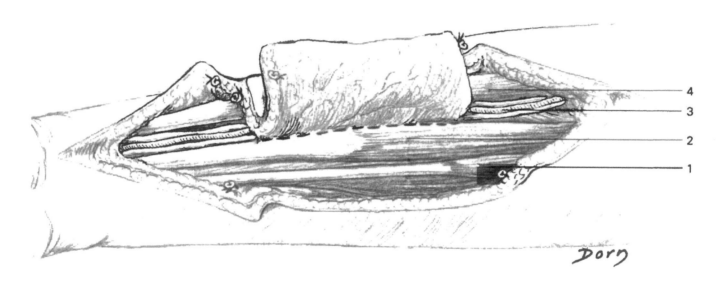

B
1 brachioradialis
2 radial nerve (sensitive branch)
3 extensor carpi radialis longus
4 flexor carpi radialis
5 palmaris longus

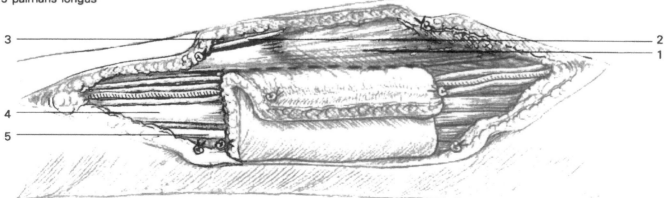

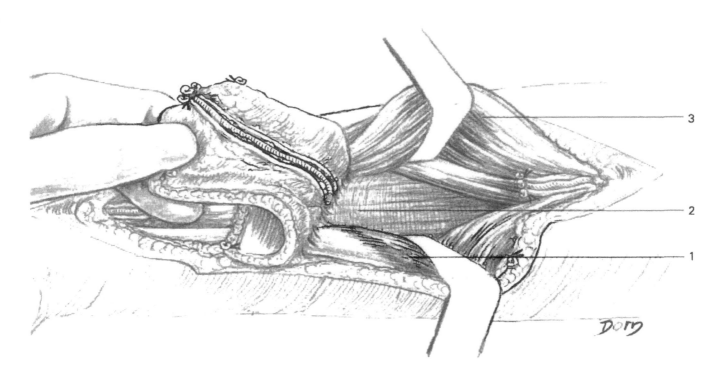

C   The radial artery has been severed proximal to
the flap. The pivot point of the pedicle is at the level
of the wrist. The flap is convenient for covering any
defect of the hand.

C
1 flexor carpi radialis
2 flexor digitorum superficialis
3 brachioradialis

Reconstructive surgery

Posterior interosseous flap

The flap is raised on the posterior aspect of the forearm. The advantage of this flap is the absence of sacrifice of a main vascular axis, since it is supplied by a small artery called the posterior interosseous artery. The technique is not easy and it is difficult to represent by drawings because of the different planes of perspective in depth.

A The flap is partially raised; a posterior hinge is maintained while exploring the vessels.

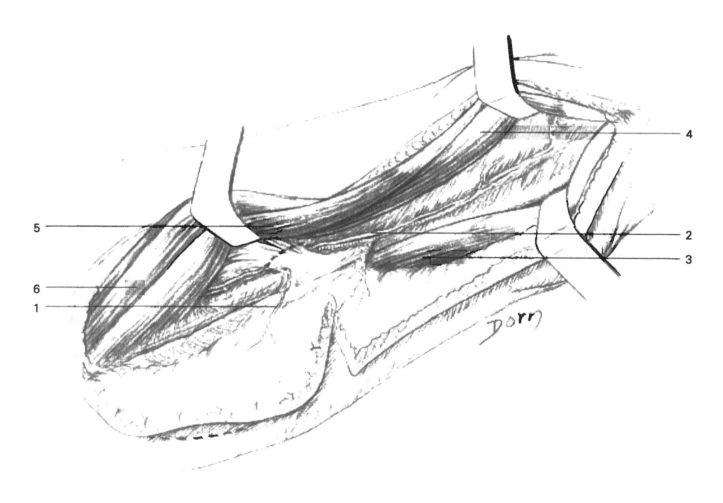

1 arterial branch to the flap
2 posterior interosseous artery
3 extensor carpi ulnaris
4 extensor indicis propius
5 extensor digiti quinti
6 extensor digitorum

B The artery is severed proximal to the branch supplying the flap. Note that the divisions of the posterior motor branch of the radial nerve are at risk during this dissection.

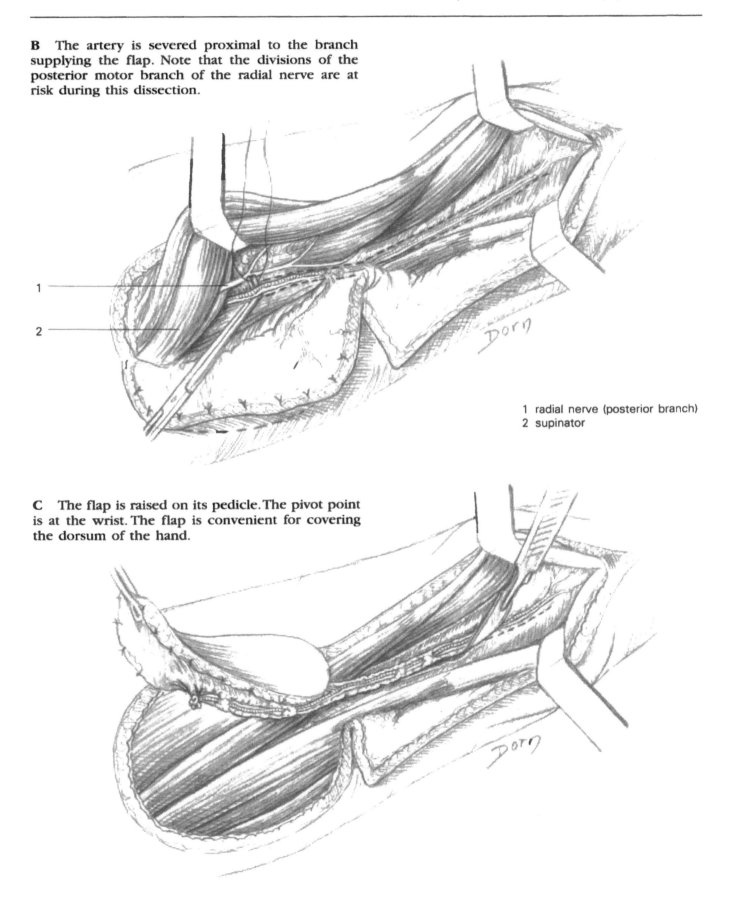

1 radial nerve (posterior branch)
2 supinator

C The flap is raised on its pedicle. The pivot point is at the wrist. The flap is convenient for covering the dorsum of the hand.

Reconstructive surgery

Pronator quadratus muscle flap

This flap is rarely used. However, the dissection is very fine and so are the drawings.

A Skin incision.

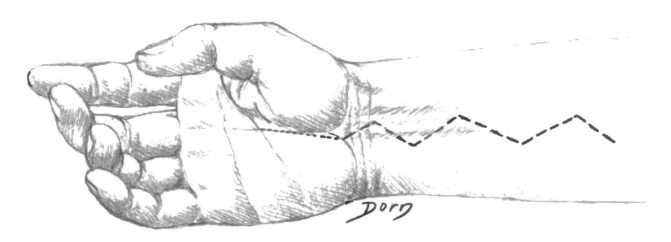

B Exposure of the pronator quadratus muscle.

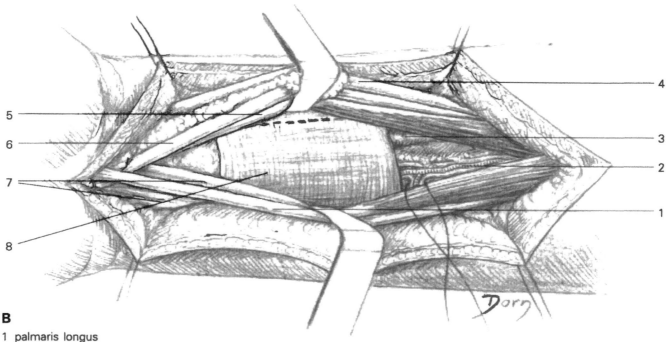

B

1 palmaris longus
2 anterior interosseous vessels
3 radius
4 flexor carpi radialis
5 flexor hallucis longus
6 median nerve
7 flexor digitorum superficialis
8 pronator quadratus

C   The flap is raised on the anterior interosseous artery.

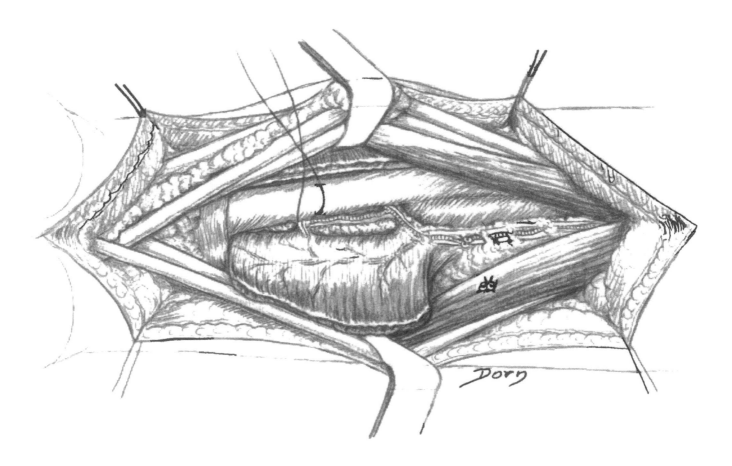

2

Hand and peripheral nerve surgery

The hand is probably a field of predilection for Léon Dorn. He has worked very hard as the hand is not easy to depict. Dorn was the renowned collaborator of Raoul Tubiana for the monumental book *Chirurgie de la Main*.

Among Dorn's vast production of illustrations of the hand can be seen some which truly demonstrate the true skill of the artist.

Anatomy of the hand

A Allen's test – the principle is to assess the permeability (patency test) of each artery of the hand.

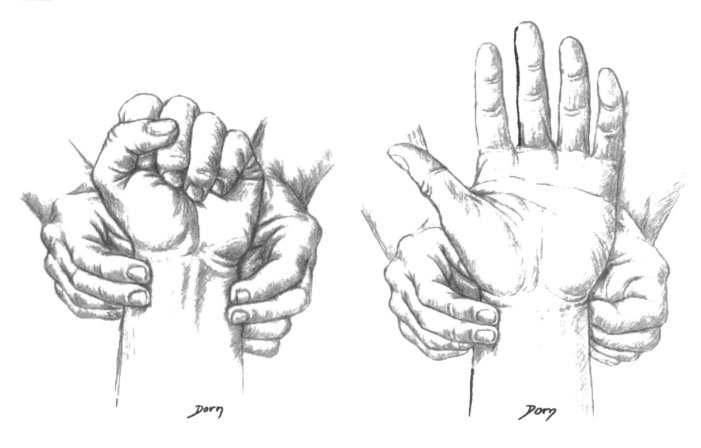

B The radial aspect of the wrist and forearm. Note the divisions of the sensory branch of the radial nerve.

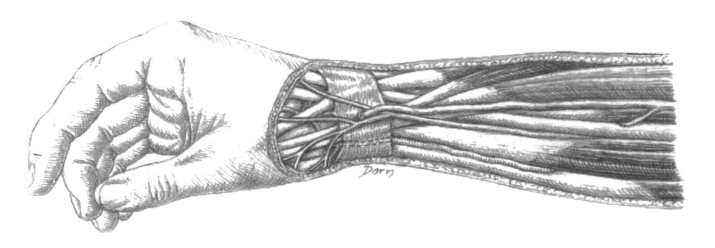

C Blood supply to the flexor tendons of the fingers. Note the small pedicles issuing from the collateral artery. They pass beneath the 'check reins' of the capsule of the PIP joint and divide into several branches. One branch is devoted to the vinculum.

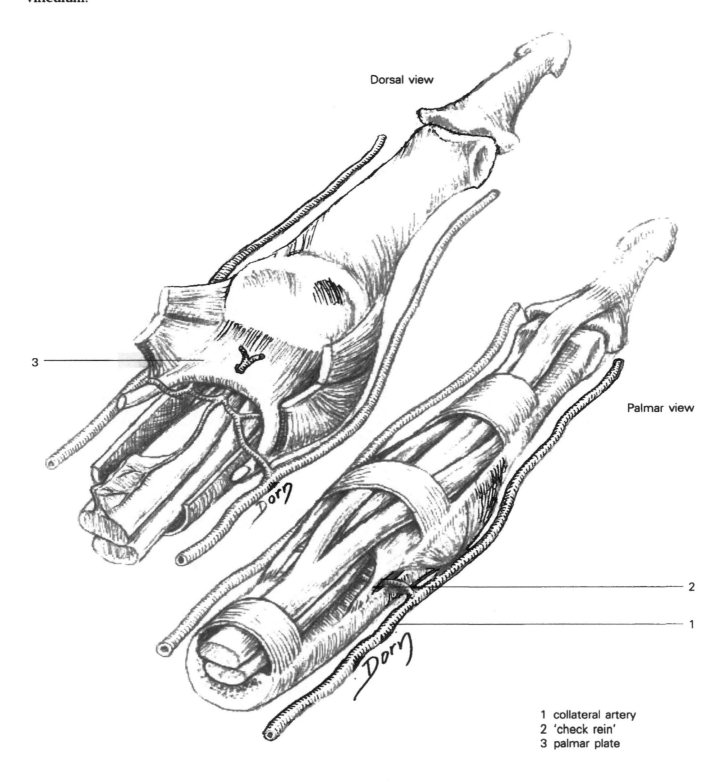

Dorsal view

Palmar view

3 palmar plate

2 'check rein'

1 collateral artery

1 collateral artery
2 'check rein'
3 palmar plate

D The blood supply to the profundus tendon comes from the vinculum of the superficialis tendon. Hence the superficialis tendon should not be excised when both tendons are divided; rather both tendons should be repaired.

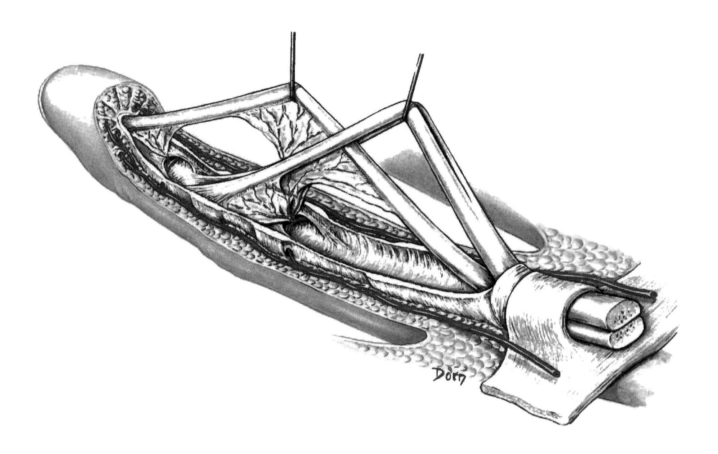

The trapezium: volar approach

The indications of this procedure are trapeziumectomy (for osteoarthritis) and internal fixation of intra-articular fractures.

A Skin incision.

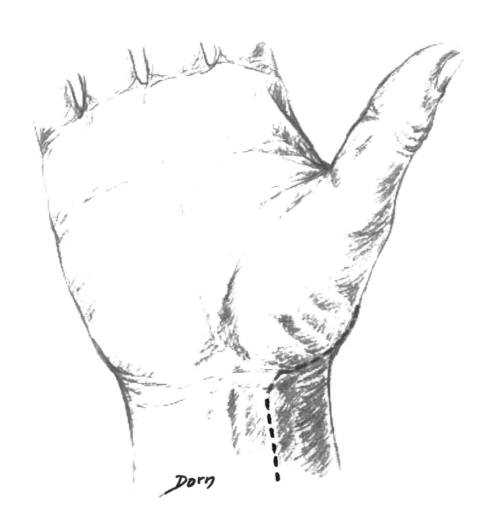

Dorn

B The muscles of the thenar eminence are reflected from the underlying capsule of the trapeziometacarpal joint.

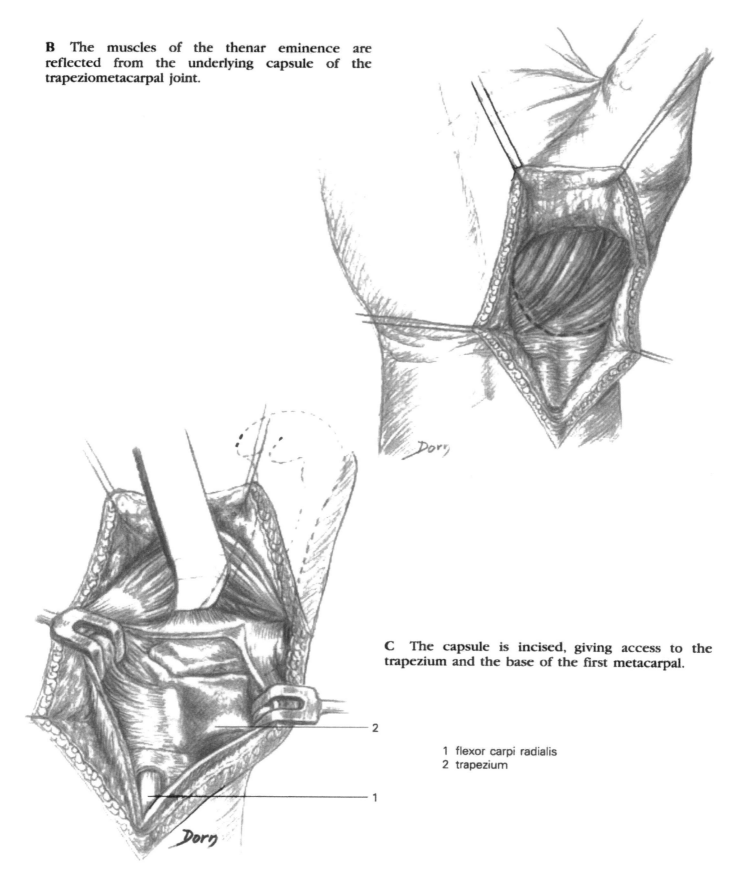

C The capsule is incised, giving access to the trapezium and the base of the first metacarpal.

1 flexor carpi radialis
2 trapezium

D, E The trapezium has been removed. A band of tendon from the flexor carpi radialis is prepared to stabilise the first metacarpal bone and to fill the cavity.

D

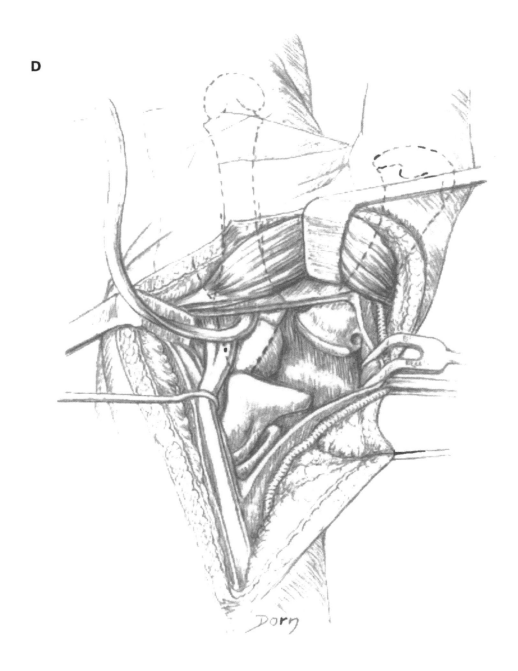

Dorn

E

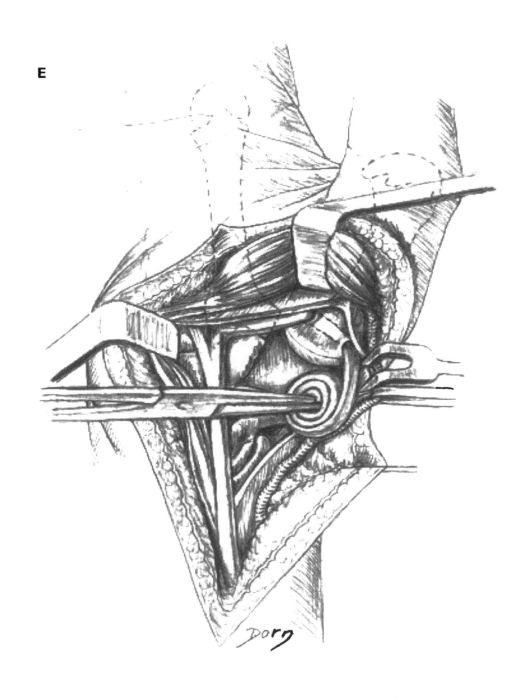

The 'boutonnière' deformity

The 'boutonnière' deformity associates flexion of the PIP joint with hyperextension of the DIP joint. It is caused by the rupture of the central band of the extensor tendon and the luxation of the lateral bands.

A Exposure of the lesions.

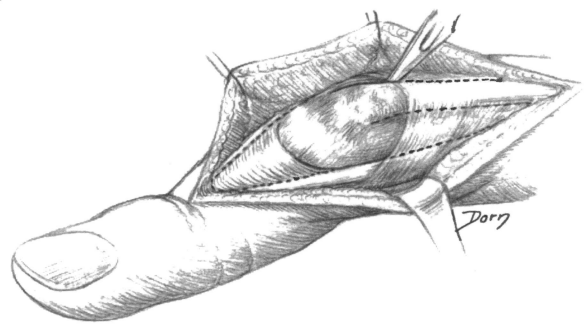

B Release of the lateral band.

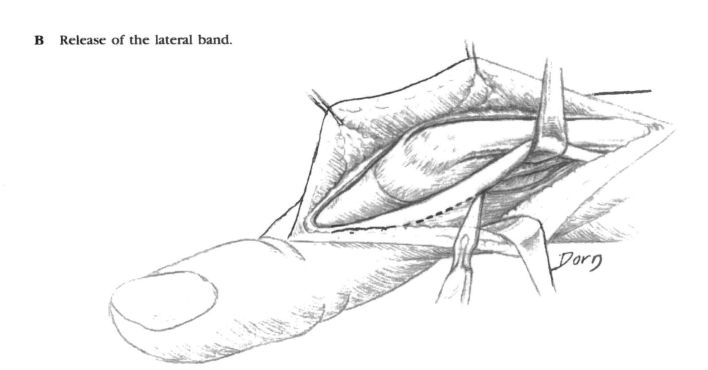

C Release of the central band.

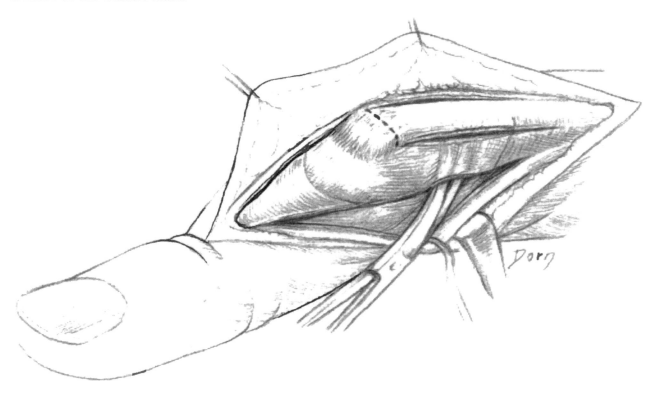

D The fibrous tissue of healing is resected to shorten the central band.

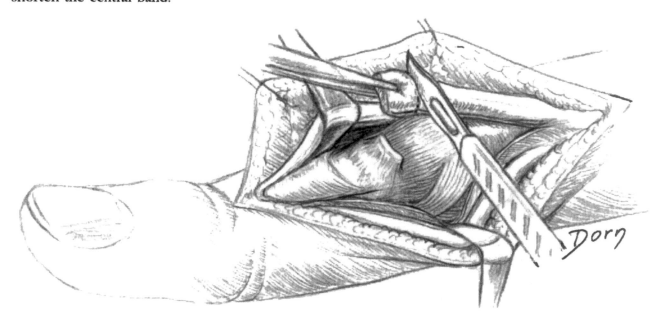

E The PIP joint is immobilised in extension with
a wire. The central band of the tendon is sutured.

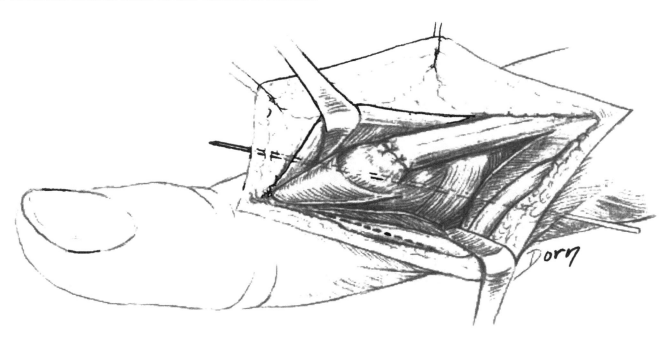

F Distal suture of the lateral bands.

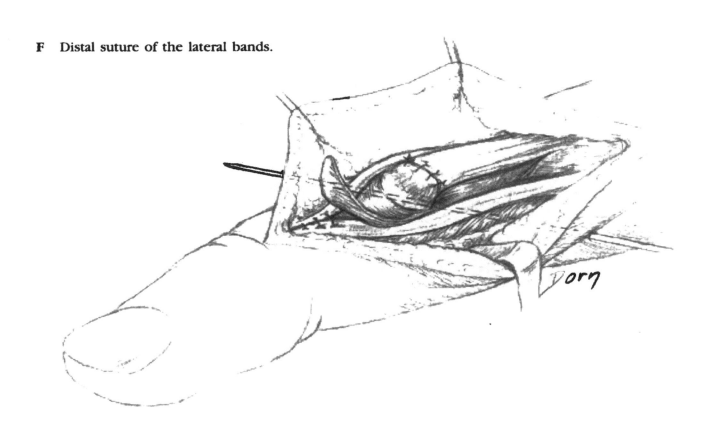

Hand and peripheral nerve surgery

Arthrolysis of the PIP joint (limitation of extension)

A The cruciate pulley of the sheath is incised and reflected.

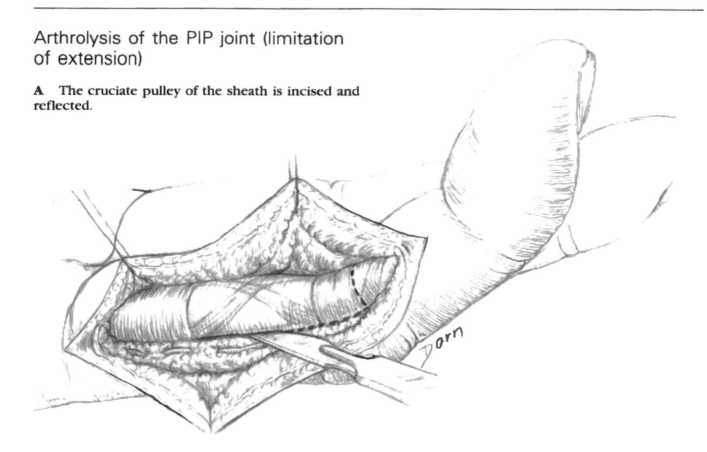

B The vincula of the flexor superficialis are well seen. The blood supply is provided by a small artery which courses just beneath the 'check rein' of the capsule.

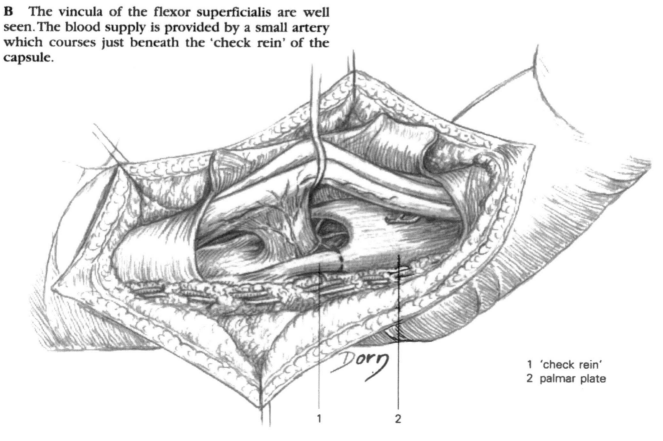

1 'check rein'
2 palmar plate

C The check rein is divided, taking care of the small artery. This constitutes the first step of the arthrolysis, and most of the time this is sufficient. If it is not, the capsule is released.

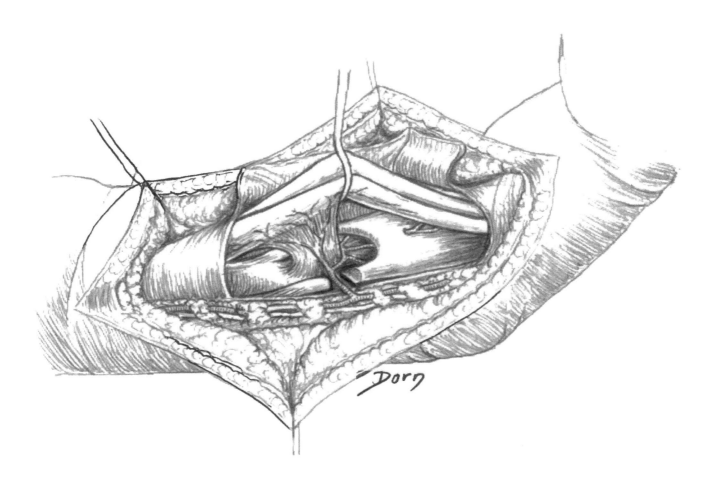

Hand and peripheral nerve surgery

Protective flap for the median nerve at the wrist

This procedure is indicated in iterative release of the median nerve in carpal tunnel syndrome.

A The fat pad of Guyon's compartment is mobilised. It is supplied by the ulnar artery.

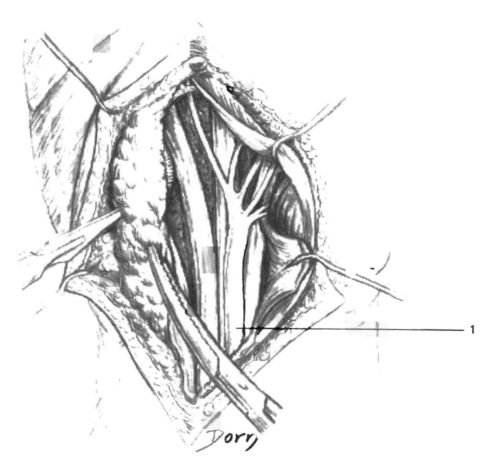

1 median nerve

B The fat flap is turned like a page of a book to cover the median nerve.

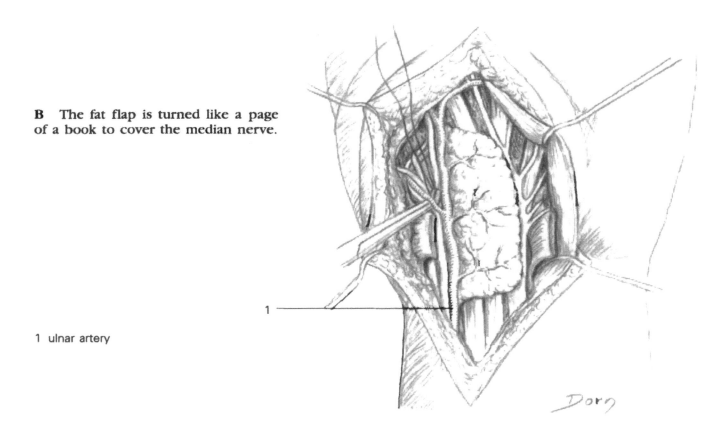

1 ulnar artery

C If necessary, the ulnar vessels are mobilised to increase the arc of rotation of the flap.

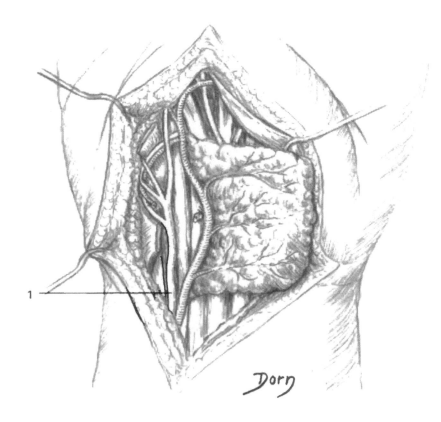

1 ulnar nerve

Flexor digitorum superficialis transfer to the thumb

This procedure allows, in a single drawing, to see the opposite side of the base of the thumb. Therefore, we can see the fixation of the tendon transfer on the ulnar side of the thumb.

Paralysis of all intrinsic muscles of the thumb. FDS transfer to the thumb. The best site for the pulley is at the proximal pole of the pisiform. The simplest procedure consists of passing the transfer around the tendon of the FCU. However, if this muscle is paralysed, its tendon stretches and the direction of the transfer will not be maintained. In this event it is advisable to perform a tenodesis of the paralysed FCU tendon to the ulna proximal to the pulley.

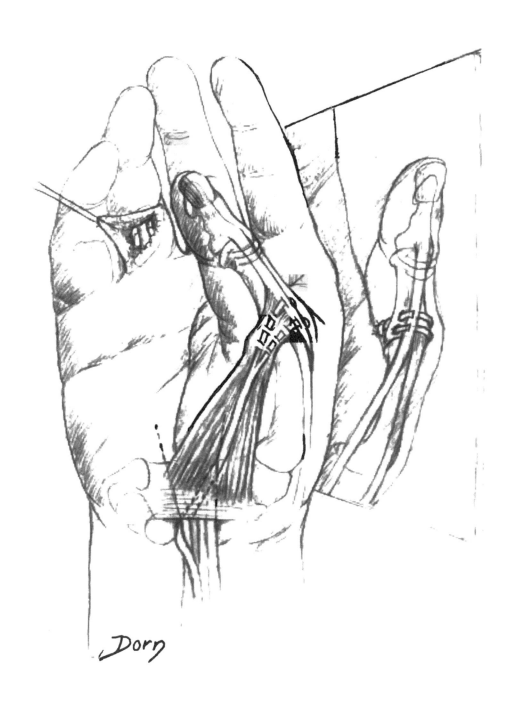

Dorn

Vascularised bone transfer from the metaphysis of the second metacarpal

The bone block is pedicled on the first dorsal interosseous artery. This transfer can be used for atrophic non-union of the scaphoid.

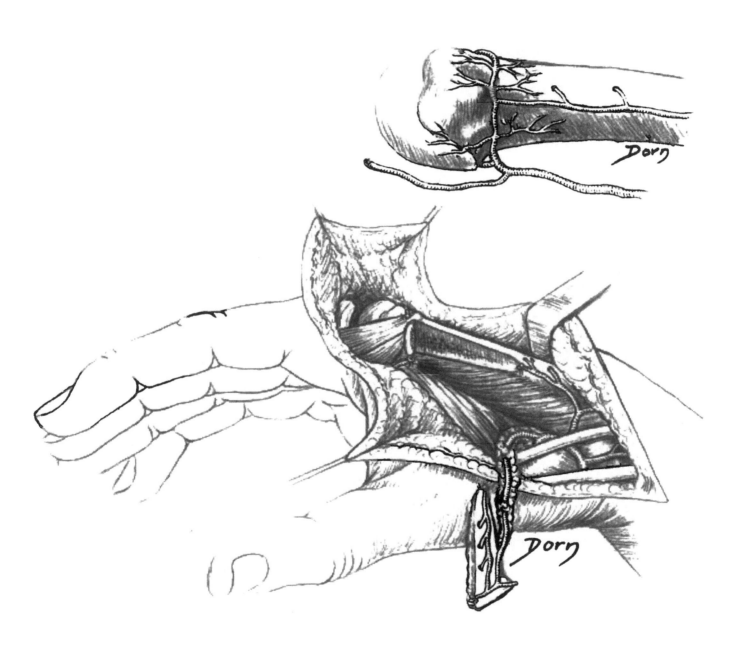

Dupuytren's disease

This series of illustrations is probably one of the most beautiful of all of Léon Dorn's drawings. The amount of work needed for representing the lesions is impressive. The drawings are based on the vast experience of Raoul Tubiana, and the fibrous bands are not a product of imagination.

A Radial side lesions.

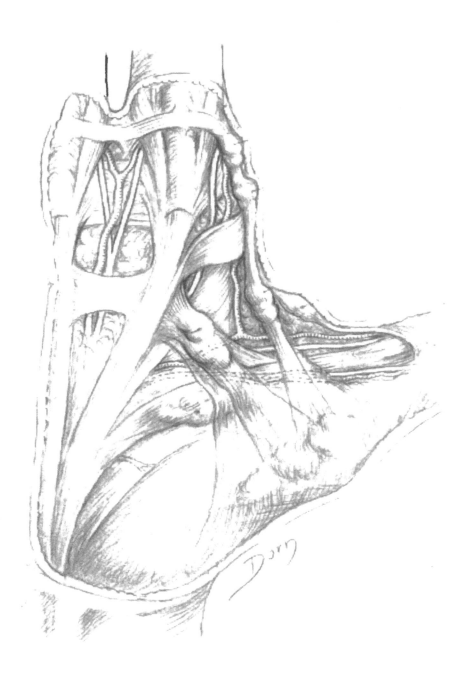

B At the digitopalmar junction and in the finger, pathological tissue is often very thick. It is necessary to identify the arteries and nerves at the level of the finger.

1 radial collateral nerve of the thumb
2 ulnar vascular bundle of the thumb
3 radial collateral nerve of the index finger

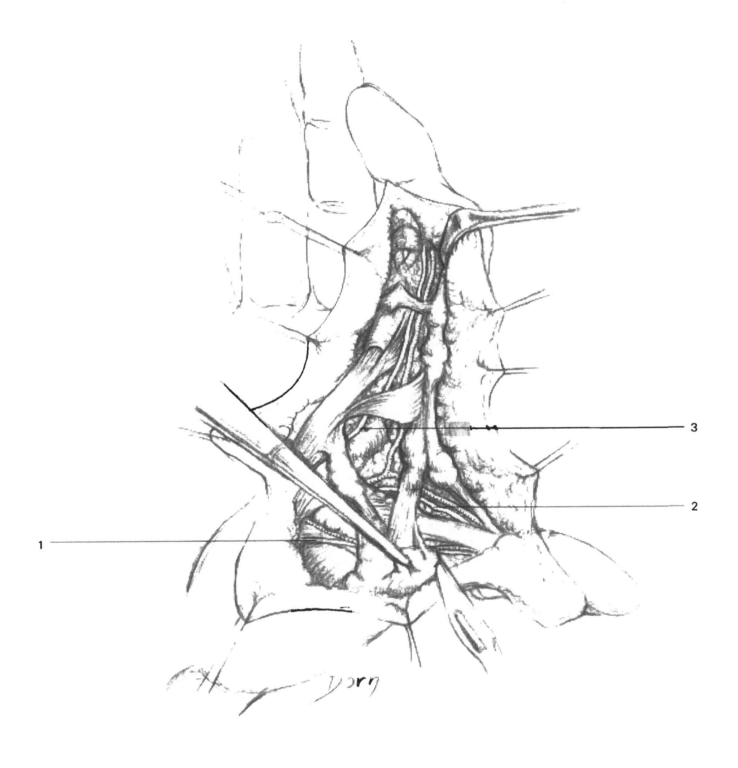

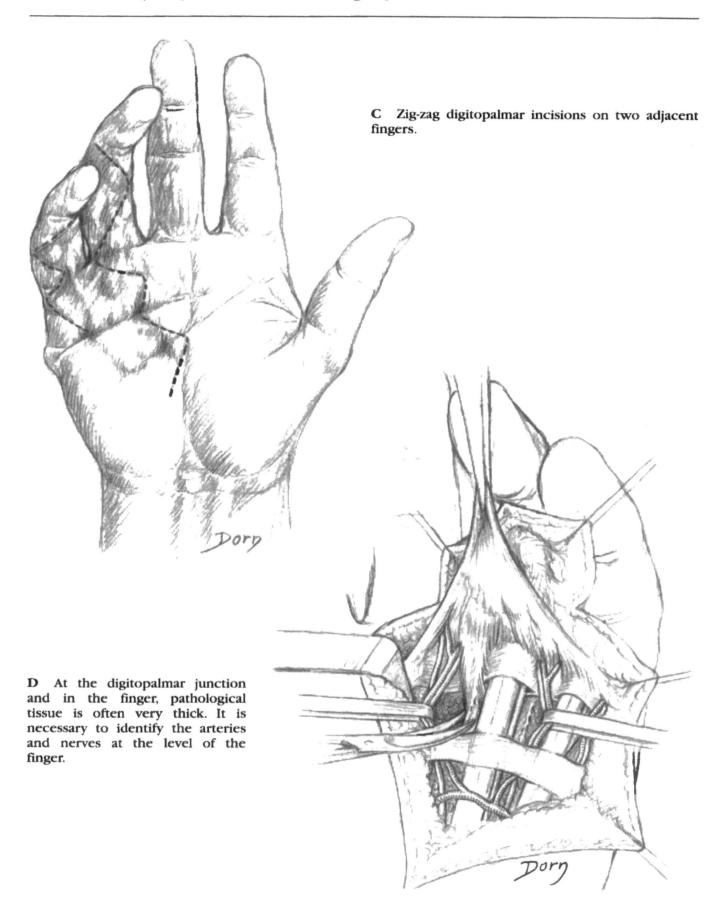

C Zig-zag digitopalmar incisions on two adjacent fingers.

D At the digitopalmar junction and in the finger, pathological tissue is often very thick. It is necessary to identify the arteries and nerves at the level of the finger.

E   Division of the vertical septae.

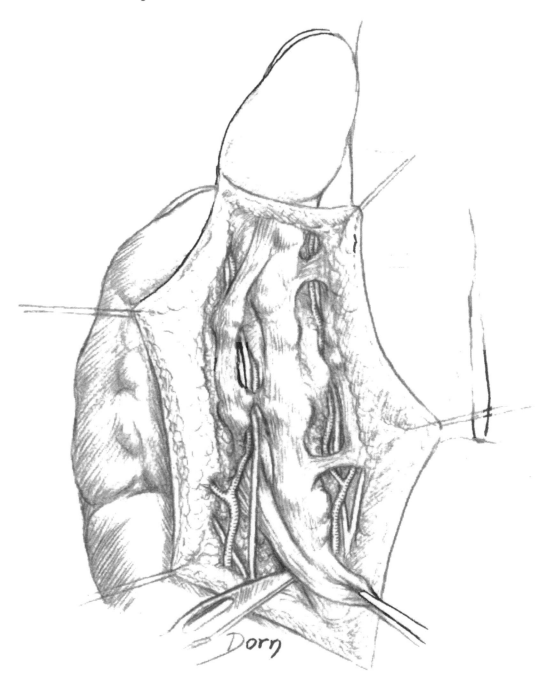

Surgery of the wrist

Approach to the distal radioulnar joint.

A The fifth compartment of extensor tendons has been opened. The tendon of extensor digit minimi is retracted and the floor of the sheath is incised.

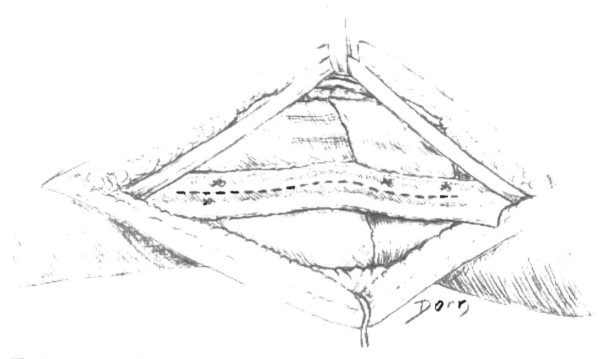

B The joint is exposed. Note rupture of the posterior radioulnar ligament.

1 ulnar head
2 radioulnar ligament

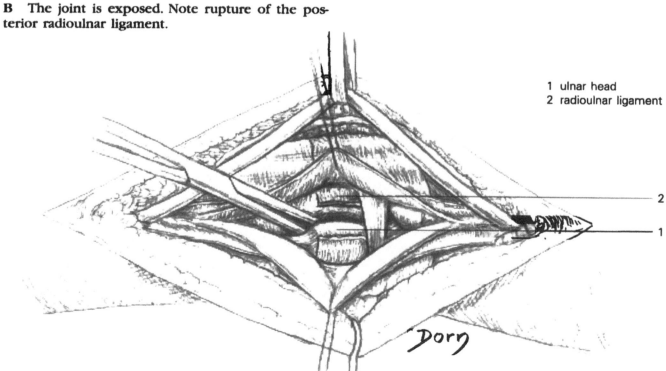

Pollicisation of the index finger

The procedure of pollicisation consists of transferring a finger to replace a missing thumb. It is one of the most difficult techniques in surgery of the hand. The skin incision should be precisely designed, dissection must be accurate and cautious and the result should be assessed cosmetically and functionally. The series of drawings shows pollicisation of the index finger, which is the most frequently performed.

A Dissection of the dorsal aspect, skin flaps being reflected.

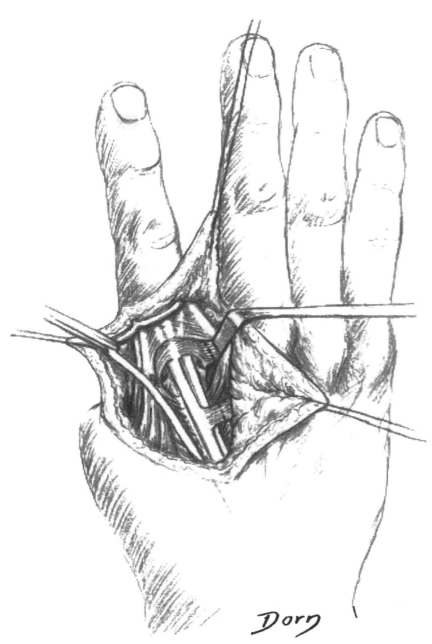

Dorn

B   Dissection of the palmar structures. Care should be taken to spare the neurovascular pedicles. Note that the common digital nerve should be split (by intraneural dissection) to allow the mobilisation of the finger.

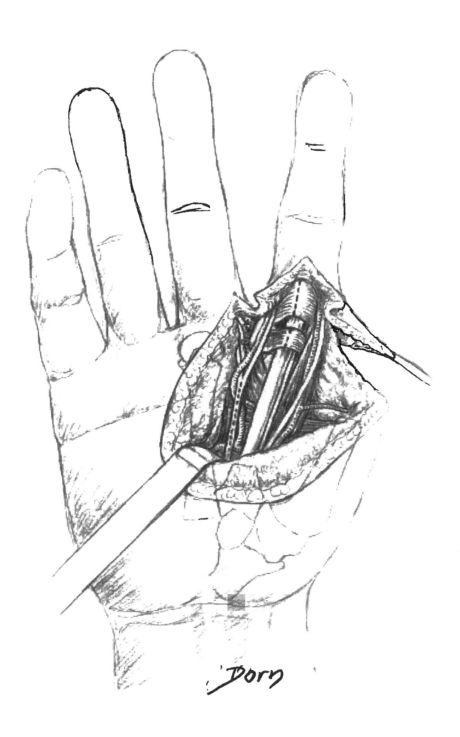

C The finger remains pedicled only on its neurovascular bundles: palmar pedicles and dorsal vein. The tendons are severed to be sutured on the recipient site. The index finger should be rotated without twisting the pedicles. Note that the first phalanx has been removed.

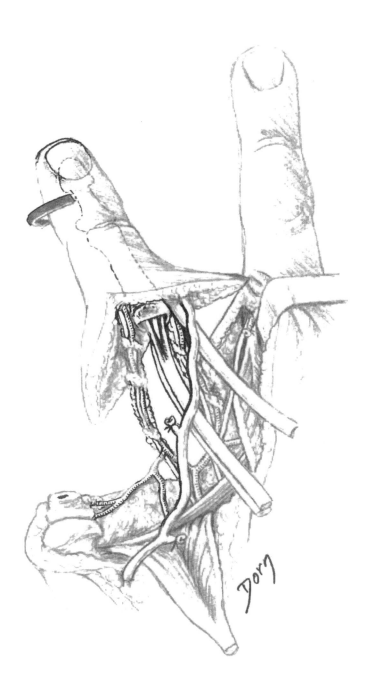

D Fixation of bone and sutures of the tendons. The second metacarpal has been excised to increase the width of the first web.

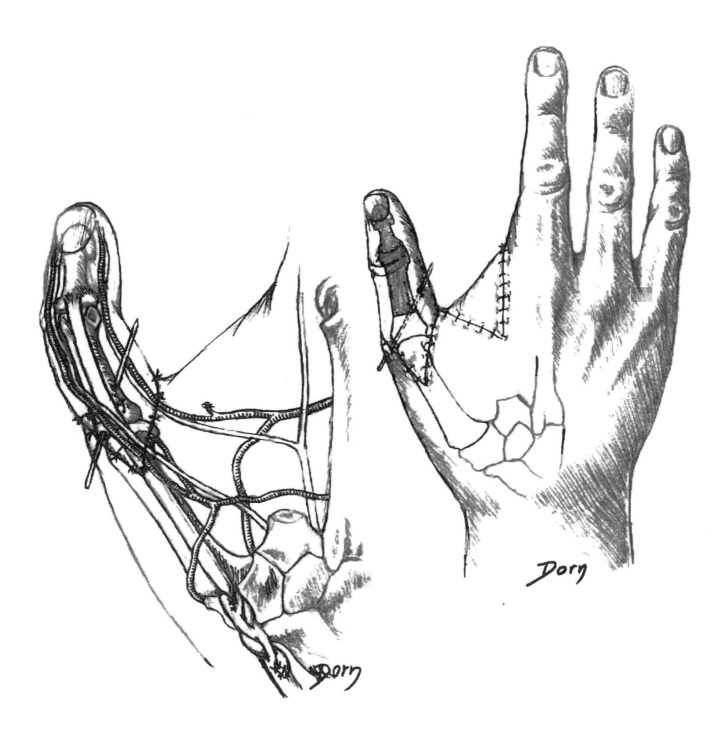

Surgery of the peripheral nerves

Nerve surgery is particularly important in the upper limb, as the ultimate purpose of the upper extremity is the function of the hand. Tunnel syndromes are frequent (median nerve at the wrist, ulnar nerve at the elbow, etc) and cause pain and disability. Traumatic lesions require exploration and repair either by direct suturing or by nerve grafts. One of the most dramatic lesions is the partial or total paralysis of the brachial plexus as a result of trauma. The first figure shows the exposure of the brachial plexus.

Brachial plexus

A, B Supraclavicular approach. The two drawings show the progressive dissection to the plexus, severing the omohyoideus (a) and then the scalenus anterior (b). Note the coloured neurovascular structures which form a key point for the rough drawings.

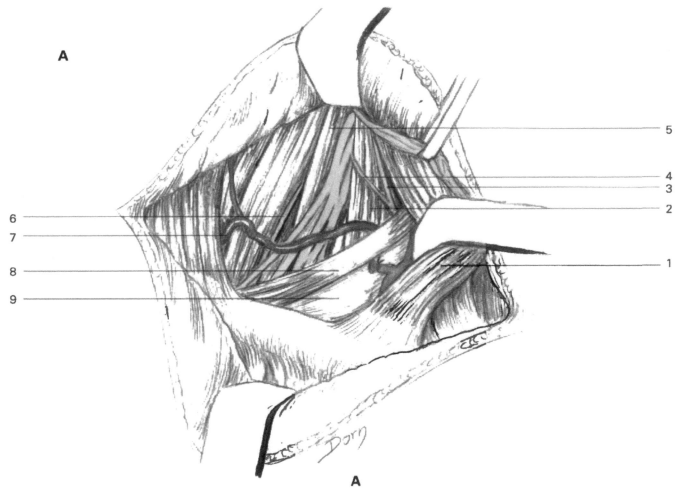

A

1 retracted sternocleidomastoid
2 scalenus anterior
3 phrenic nerve
4 accessory phrenic nerve
5 scalenus medius
6 branch to rhomboid and levator scapular
7 superficial cervical artery
8 omohyoideus
9 omohyoideus fascia

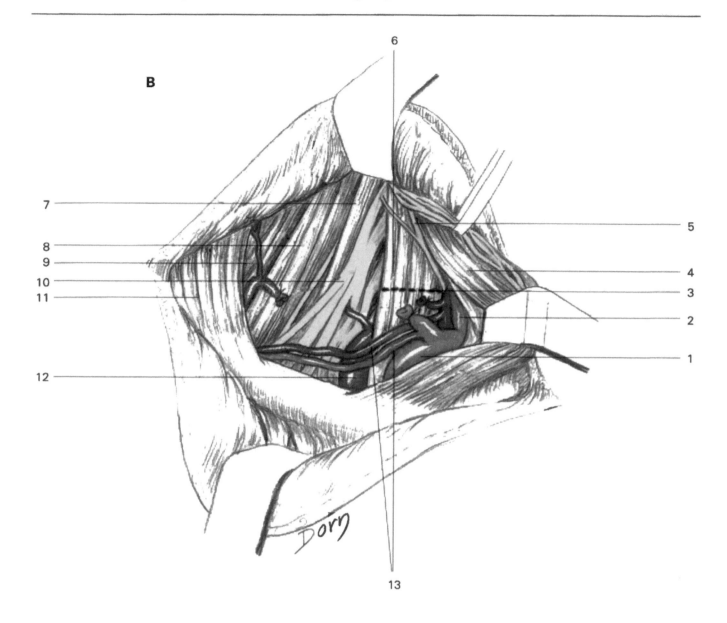

B

1 subclavian vein
2 int. jugular vein
3 line of division of scalenus ant.
4 sterno-cleidomastoid retracted
5 phrenic nerve retracted
6 scalenus anterior
7 scalenus medius
8 levator scapula
9 splenius capitis
10 brachial plexus
11 trapezius
12 subclavian artery
13 supra-scapular artery and vein

C, D Supraclavicular and infraclavicular approach. Pectoralis minor is severed to expose the divisions of the plexus. If necessary the clavicle can also be osteotomised.

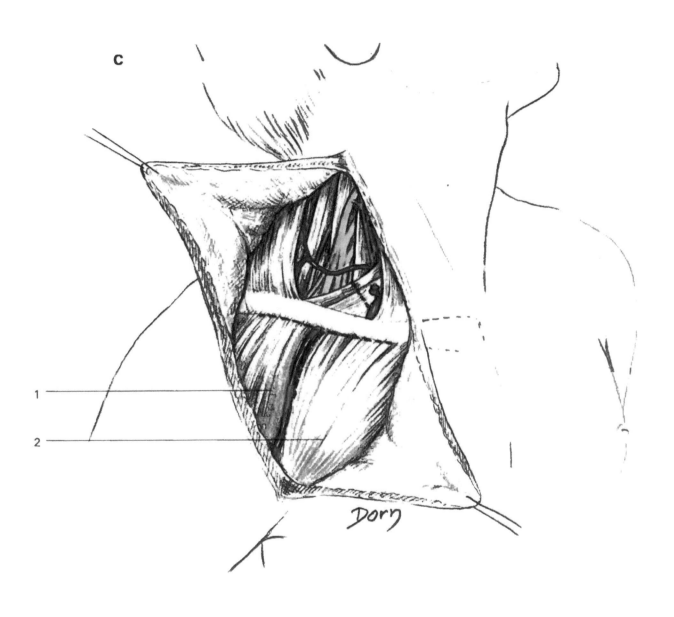

1 deltoid
2 pectoralis major

D

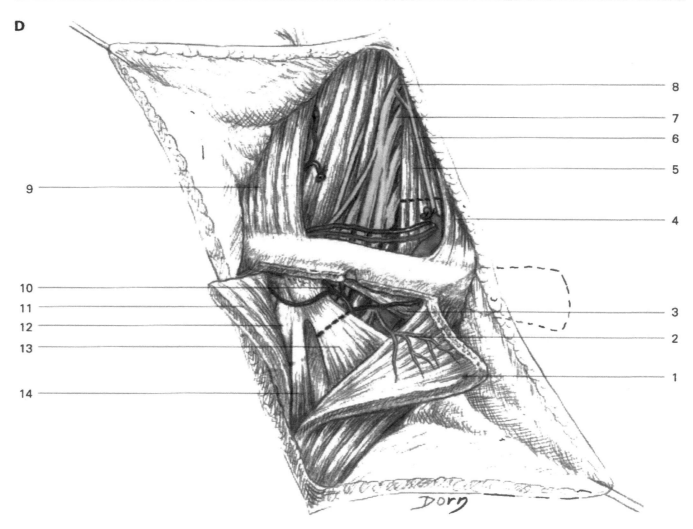

D

1 pectoralis major	5 scalenus anterior	10 thoraco-acromial artery
2 lat. pectoral nerve	6 phrenic nerve	11 deltoid
3 subclavius	7 C6	12 short head biceps
4 sterno-cleidomastoid	8 C5	13 pectoralis minor
	9 trapezius	14 coraco brachial

E

1 serratus anterior	17 C7	33 nerve to coracobrachialis
2 pectoralis major	18 phrenic nerve	34 pectoralis major
3 pectoralis minor	19 branch to phrenic nerve	35 deltoid
4 thoracodorsal nerve	20 C6	36 median nerve
5 inferior subscapular nerve	21 C5	37 axillary nerve
6 superior subscapular nerve	22 C4	38 coracobrachialis
7 second intercostal nerve	23 accessory nerve	39 biceps brachii
8 second rib	24 branch to rhomboids	40 profunda brachii
9 long thoracic nerve	25 subclavius nerve	41 axillary artery
10 subclavius muscle	26 suprascapular nerve	42 radial nerve
11 subclavian vein	27 trapezius	43 ulnar nerve
12 subclavian artery	28 acromiothoracic artery	44 axillary vein
13 T1	29 pectoralis minor	45 medial brachial vutaneous nerve of arm
14 suprascapular artery	30 upper subscapular nerve	46 latissimus dorsi
15 C8	31 cephalic vein	
16 scalenus anterior	32 musculocutaneous nerve	

E   Anatomical view of all structures.

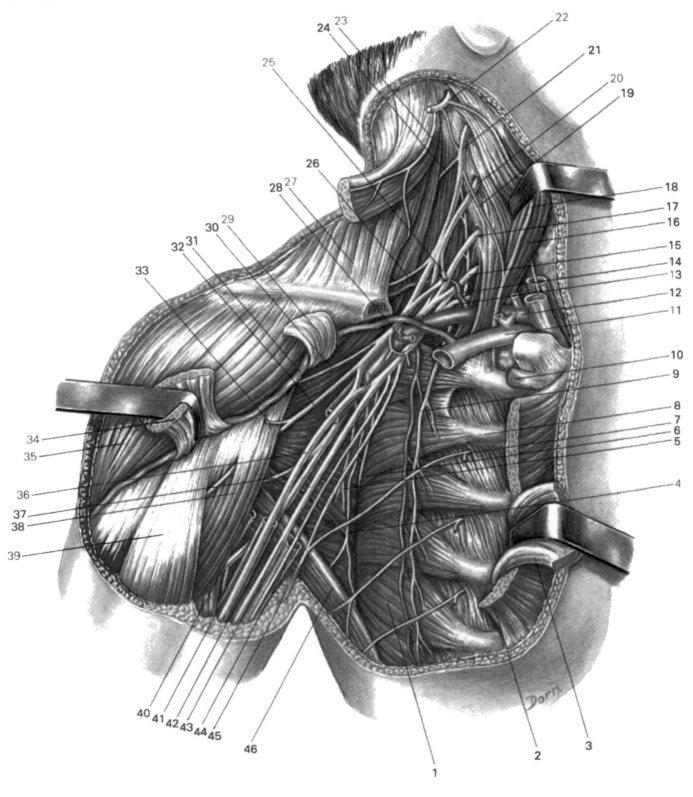

Exposure of the interosseous nerve (posterior motor branch of the radial nerve)

A Skin incision on the posterolateral aspect of the forearm.

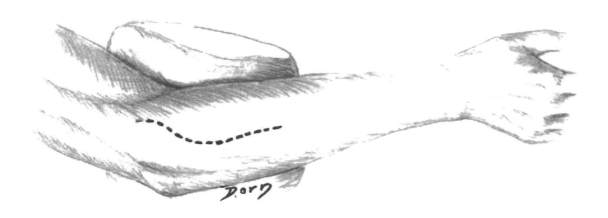

B Muscles are exposed. Two approaches are mandatory: the first one between the extensors of the carpus and the extensor digitorum communis and the second one between the extensors of the fingers and extensor carpi ulnaris.

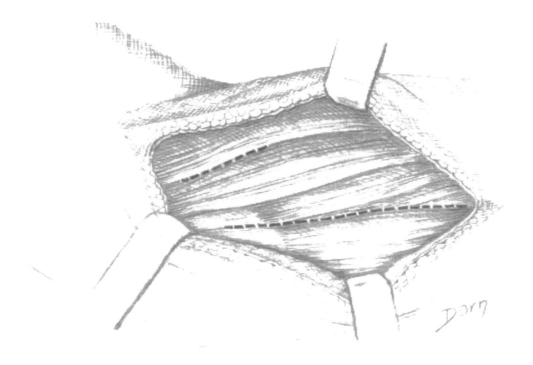

C, D The posterior radial nerve is identified proximally and distally to the supinator muscle.

C

1

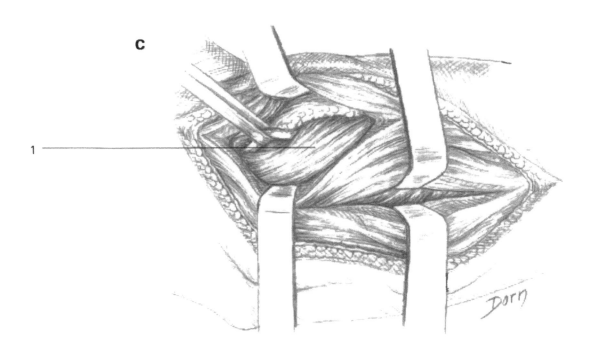

1 suprinator

D

1

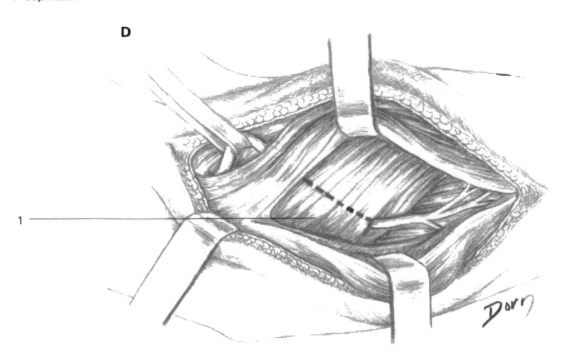

E Superficial head of the supinator has been severed to release the nerve.

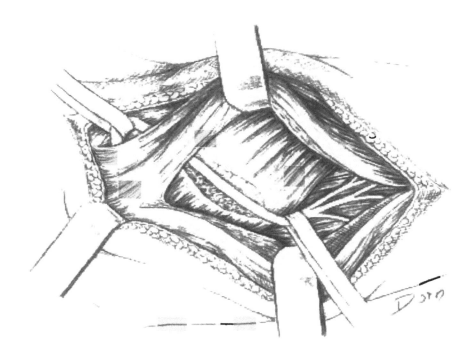

Exposure of the radial nerve at the elbow (common trunk and its division into anterior and posterior branches)

A The plane between the brachioradialis and brachialis is developed.

B Medially the biceps and the pronator teres muscles are retracted. The radial nerve and its division are exposed. The posterior branch courses beneath the superficial head of the supinator muscle.

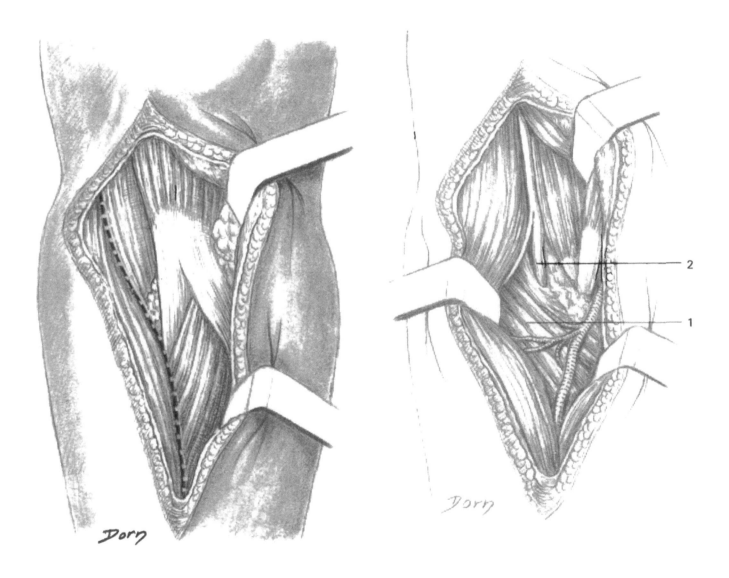

1 suprinator
2 radial nerve

C By reflecting the brachioradialis muscle, the anterior branch is exposed. It courses near the radial artery.

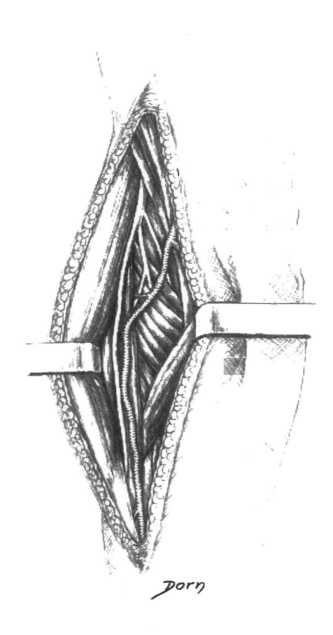

Dorn

3

Gynaecological surgery

Some of these drawings have been made from rough sketches made in the operating theatre. They illustrate the numerous techniques for treating genital prolapse.

Gynaecological surgery

The lower approach of the genital prolapse and the separation of the vagina and the bladder

A–C The anterior aspect of the vagina is incised and the plane of dissection between the vagina and the bladder is developed.

A

B

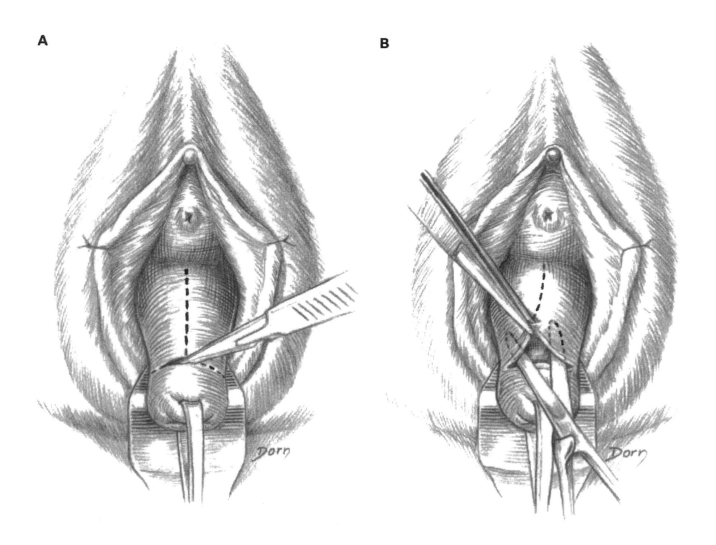

D–F The separation between the vagina and the bladder is pursued; the long forceps holds the bladder.

C

D

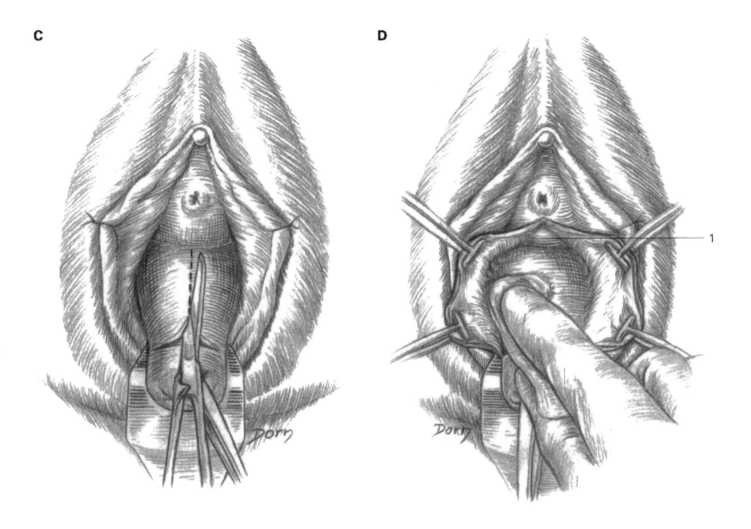

1 bladder

E

F

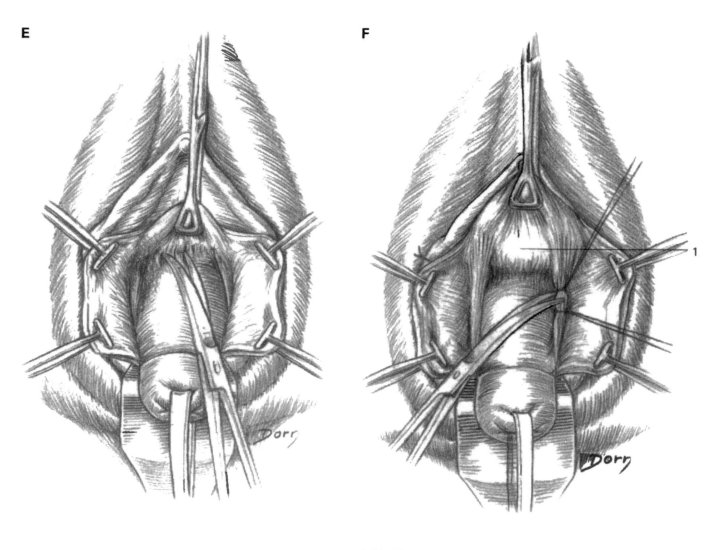

1 bladder

G, H Separation of the posterior aspect of the vagina.

G

H

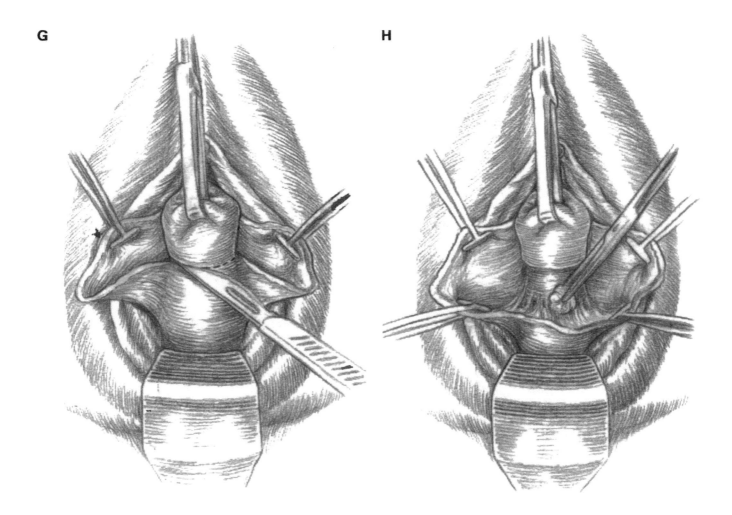

I, J The cul-de-sac of Douglas is opened and the uterosacral ligaments are ligated and cut.

I

J

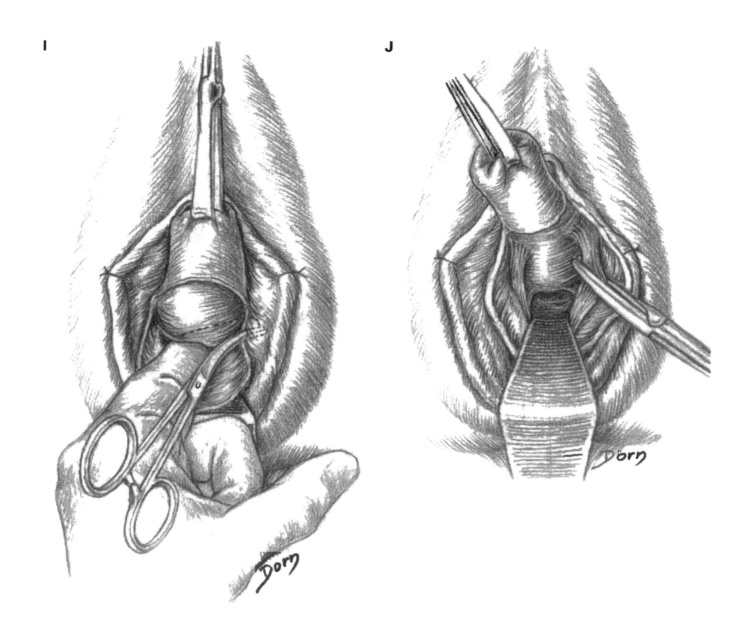

Treatment of genital prolapse after hysterectomy

A In this procedure care should be taken of the bladder which can overlap behind the cervix of the uterus (after a hysterectomy).

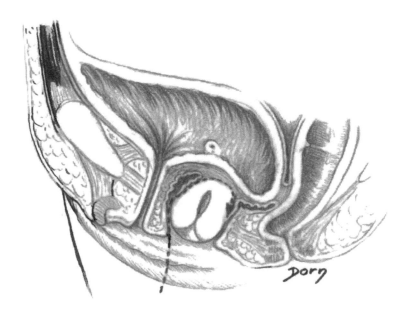

B Just before the hysterectomy, the threads are passed through the uterosacral ligaments, taking care of the ureters.

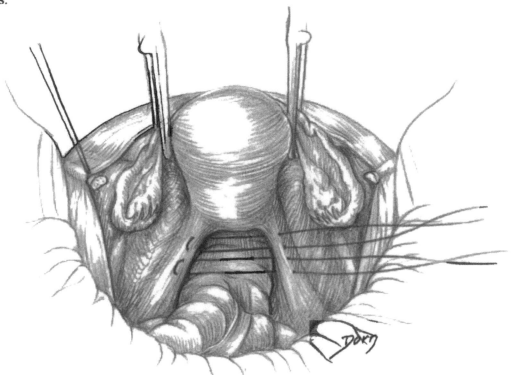

C–E The hysterectomy is completed by an upper
approach.

C

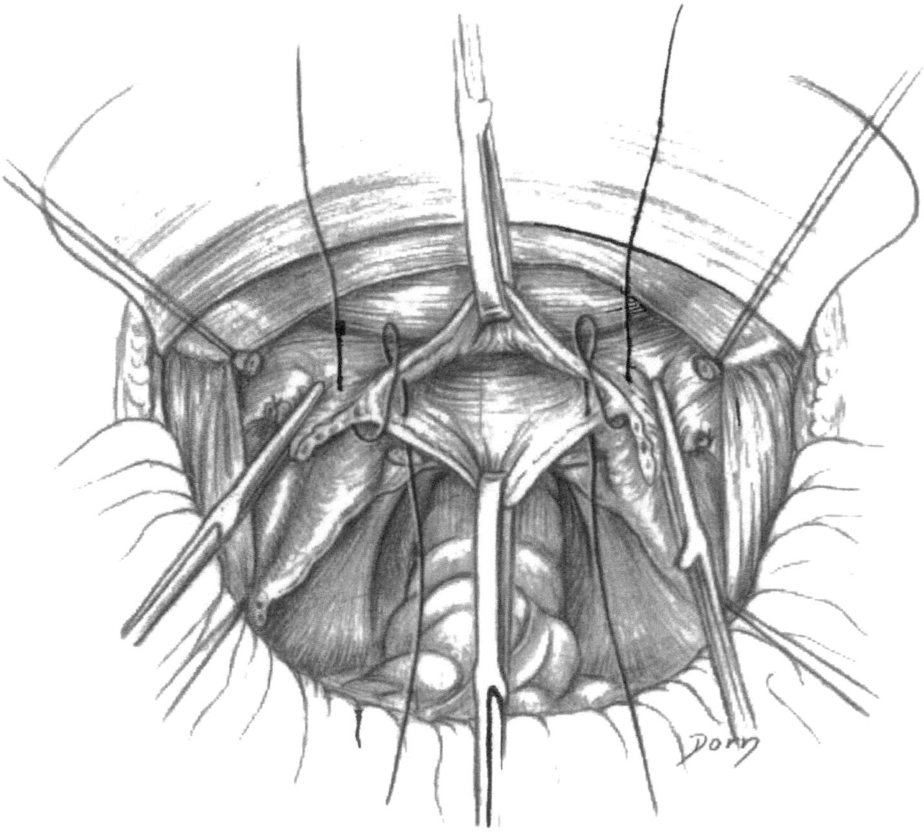

D

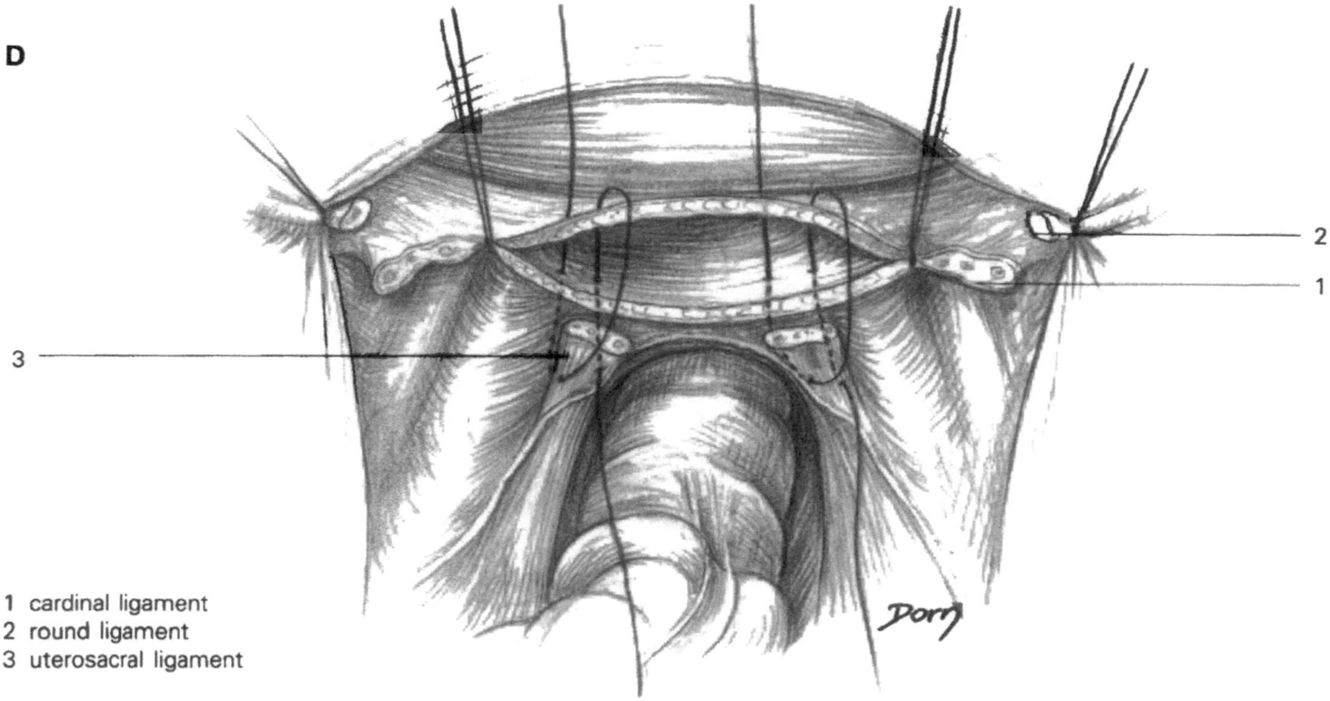

1 cardinal ligament
2 round ligament
3 uterosacral ligament

E

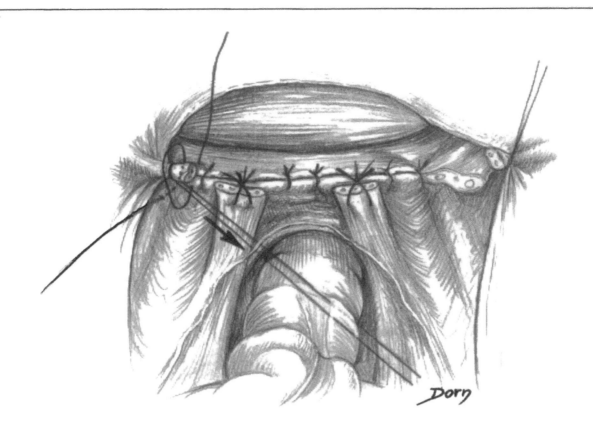

F   The vagina is sutured and the uterosacral ligaments are sutured to the vagina.

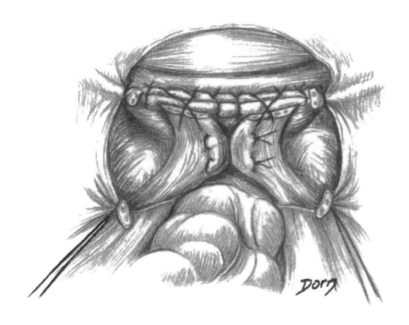

G–J The closure of the cul-de-sac of Douglas to prevent an elytrocele.

G

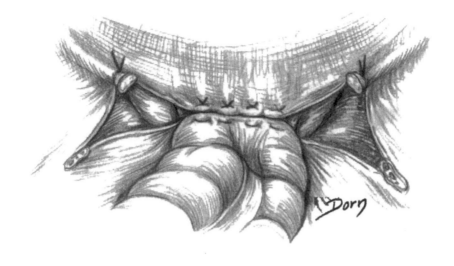

H

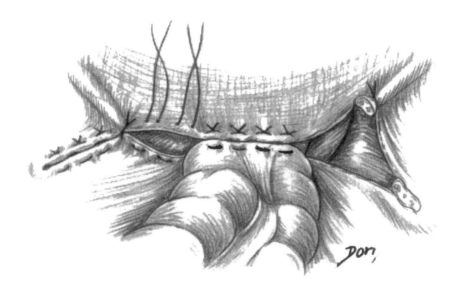

The perineum is sutured.

I

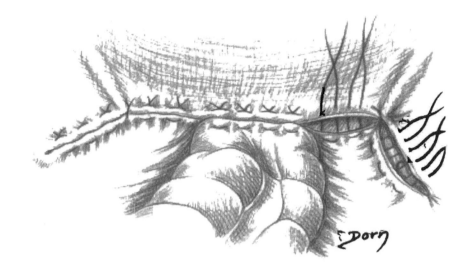

J

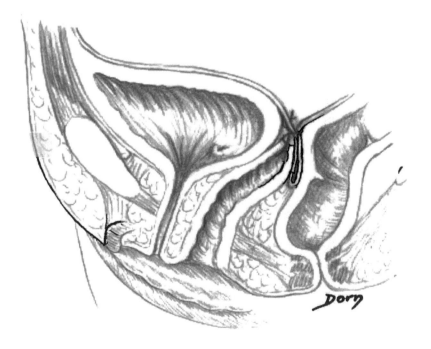

Gynaecological surgery

Surgical treatment of the elytrocele

The elytrocele is the interposition of the cul-de-sac of Douglas between the vagina and the rectum. The surgery is performed by the abdominal approach.

A The uterus is held by threads; the dotted line is the landmark for the dissection. Care should be taken to spare the ureters.

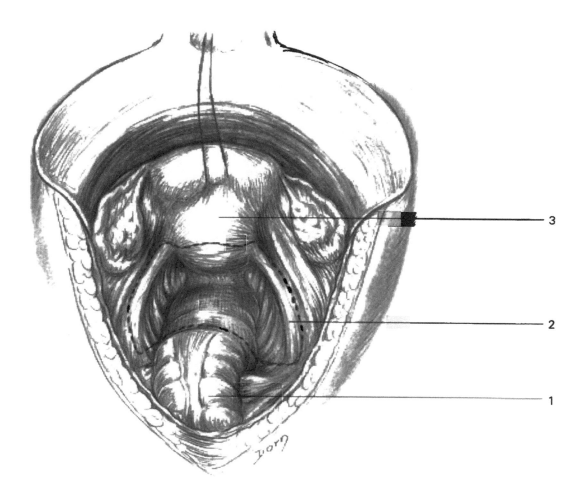

1 rectum
2 uterosacral ligament
3 uterus

B, C The plane of dissection is developed between the posterior aspect of the uterus and the rectum.

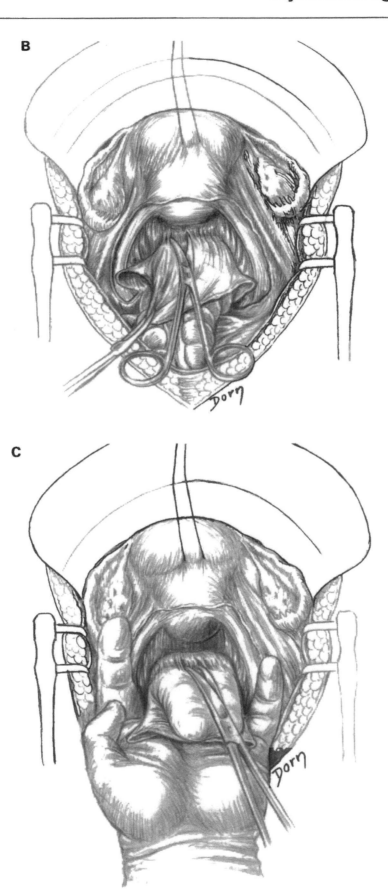

D   The uterosacral ligaments are sutured together.

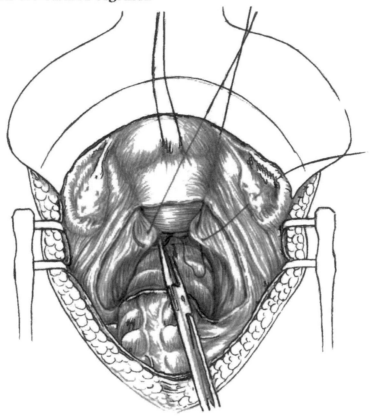

E   The peritoneum is sutured.

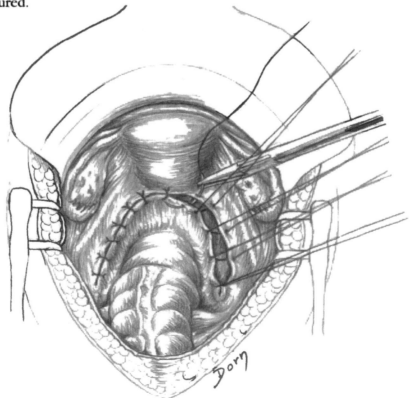

4

Urological surgery

Urology is a surgical specialty covering a large number of indications and procedures.

Transplantation of the kidney was the first successful allotransplantation to be performed a short time after the Second World War. This extraordinary achievement marked the start of the modern era of organ transplantation aided by the advances in immunology. Urology is also concerned with reconstructive procedures involving loss of substance irrespective of the aetiology: tumour, congenital, traumatic, etc.

The last section of this chapter covers surgery of the sexual organs in sex modification.

Urological surgery

Allotransplantation of the kidney

The various steps are shown in the drawings: surgical approach, preparation of the vessels and vascular anastomoses.

A Skin incision.

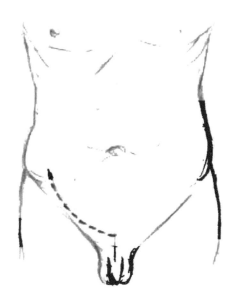

B The abdominal muscular wall is incised.

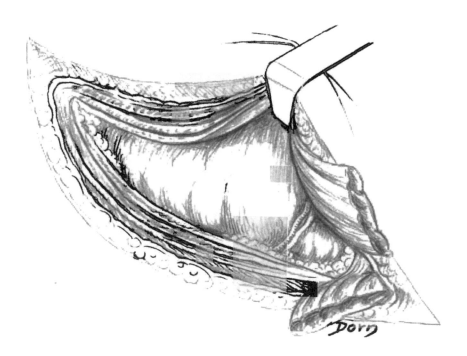

C The peritoneum is retracted which allows the dissection of the internal iliac vessels.

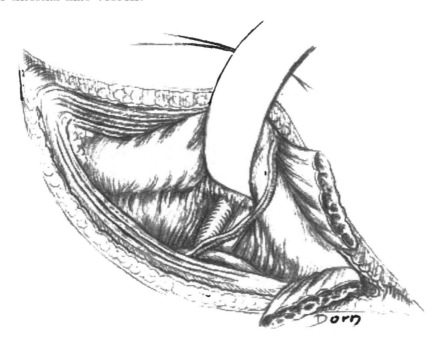

D Exposure of the division of the common iliac artery.

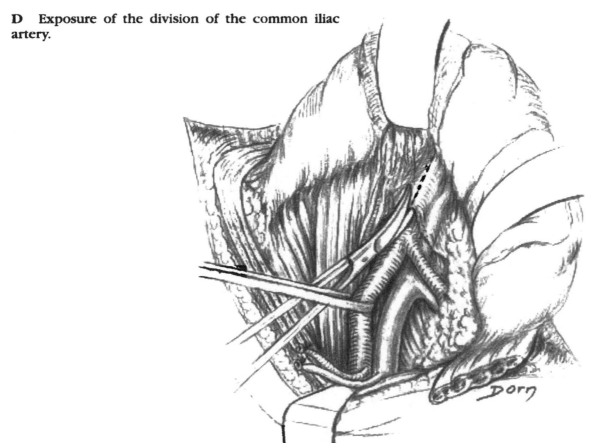

E Preparation of the recipient vein (external iliac vein).

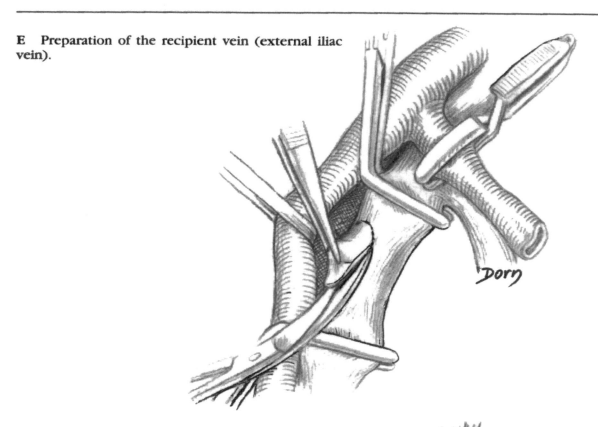

F Presentation of the transplant.

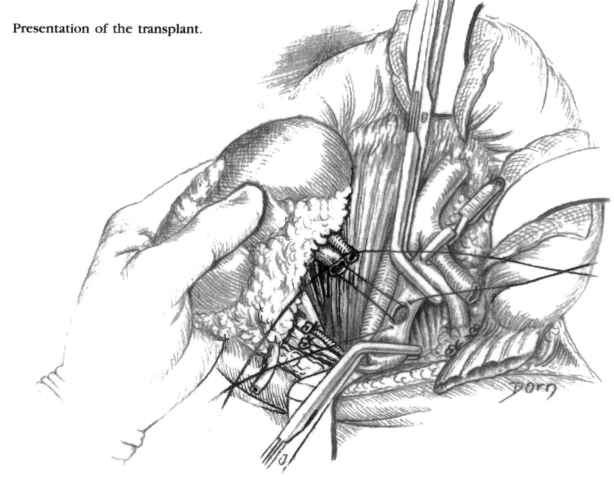

G, H Suturing the vessels. The first to be done is
the anastomosis of the veins.

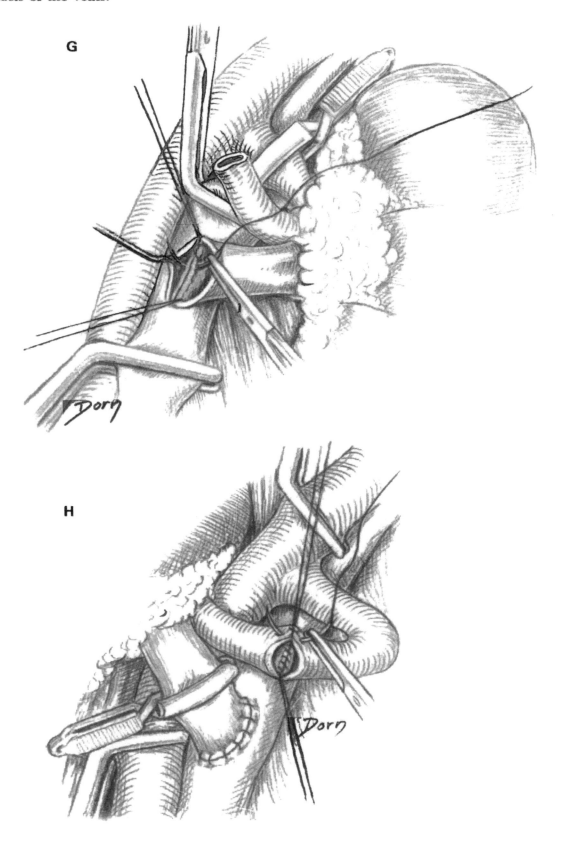

I The final aspect of the vascular sutures. Then the
ureter is reimplanted in the bladder.

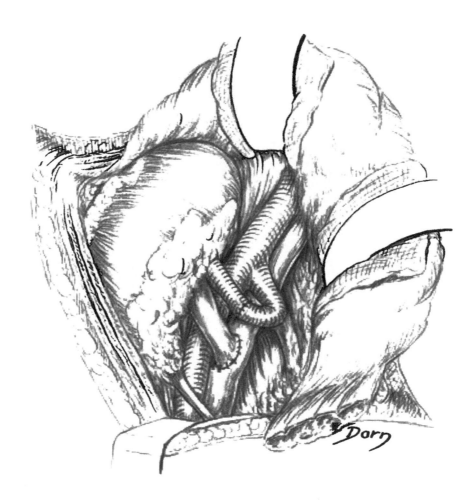

Surgery of renal lithiasis

A The compartment of the kidney has been opened. The ureter is identified.

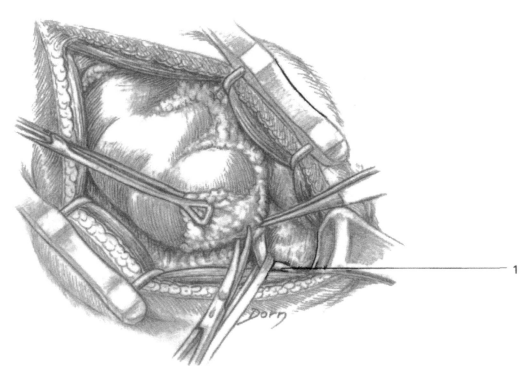

B Dissection of the ureter allows access to the renal pelvis.

1 ureter

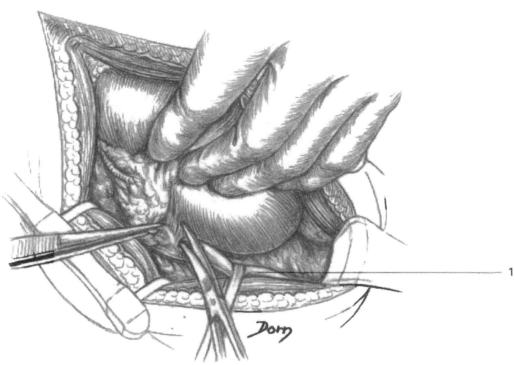

C Incision of the renal pelvis.

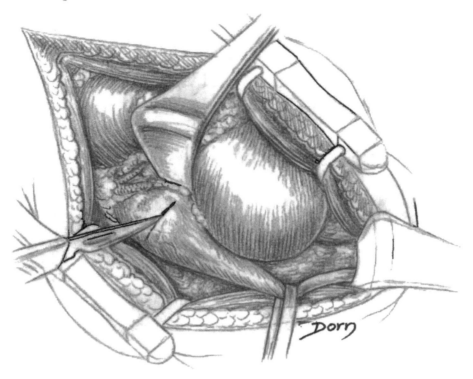

D Removing the lithiasis.

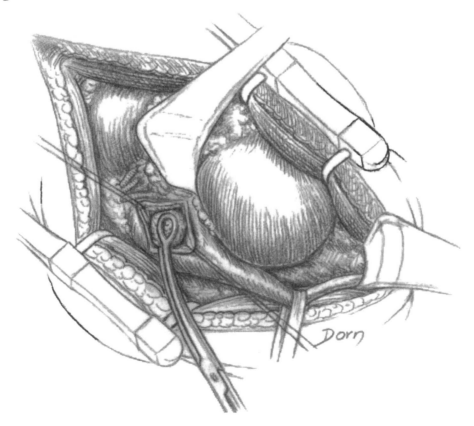

Extrophy of the bladder in a young boy

A The incisions. Two skin flaps are delineated.

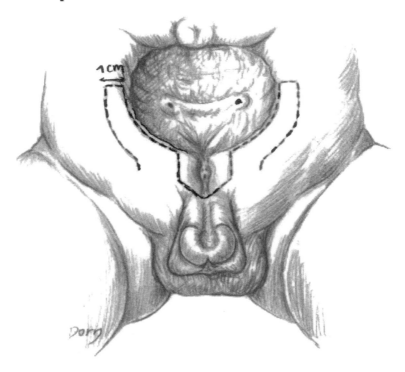

B The lateral aspects of the bladder are released.

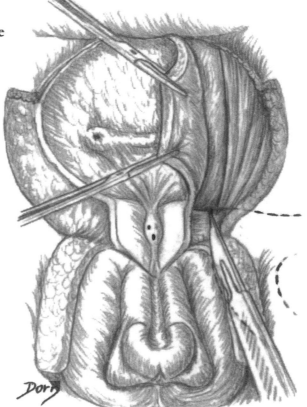

C The penis is lengthened. The ischiocavernosus muscles are released.

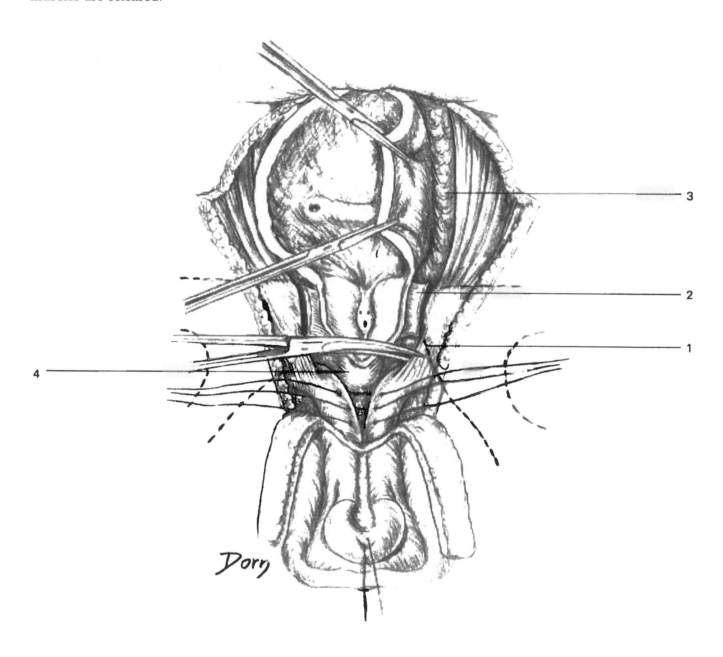

Dorr

C

1 ischiocavernosus muscle
2 transverse perineal ligament
3 release of the posterior aspect of the bladder
4 bulbospongiosus

D The urethra is lengthened by joining the two
skin flaps and the bladder is sutured.

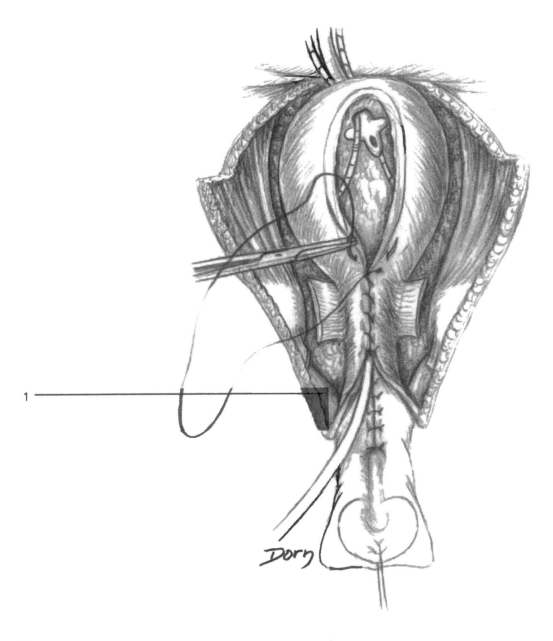

1

D

1 corpus cavernosus

E   Closure of the bone frame.

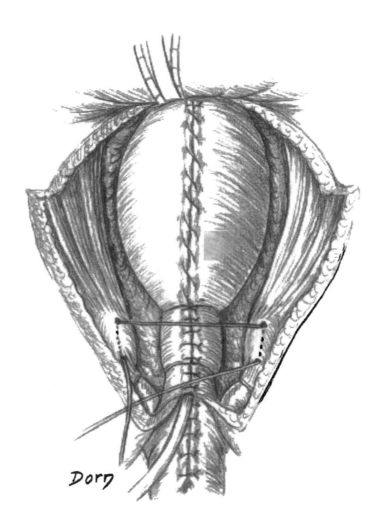

Dorn

F   Closure of the muscular wall.

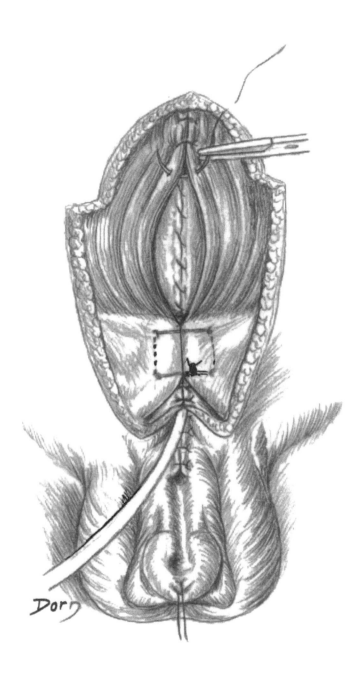

Urological surgery

Hypospadias surgery

Hypospadias is a congenital malformation in which the external urethral meatus is not contained in the glans penis.

The aim of the operation is to reconstruct the distal portion of the urethra.

A The urethral canal will be reconstructed with a tubularised and pedicled preputial flap (mucosal aspect). Design of the incisions.

B Incision around the urethral meatus.

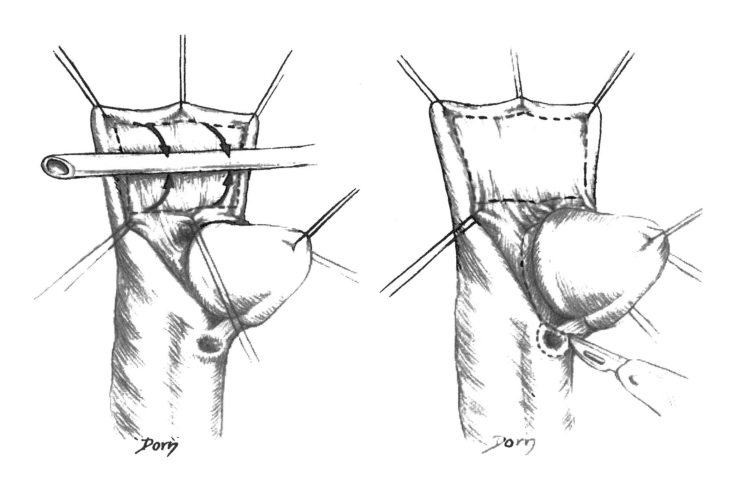

C Section of the retractile band responsible for the curvature of the penis.

D Release of the urethra between the corpora cavernosa and the corpus spongiosum.

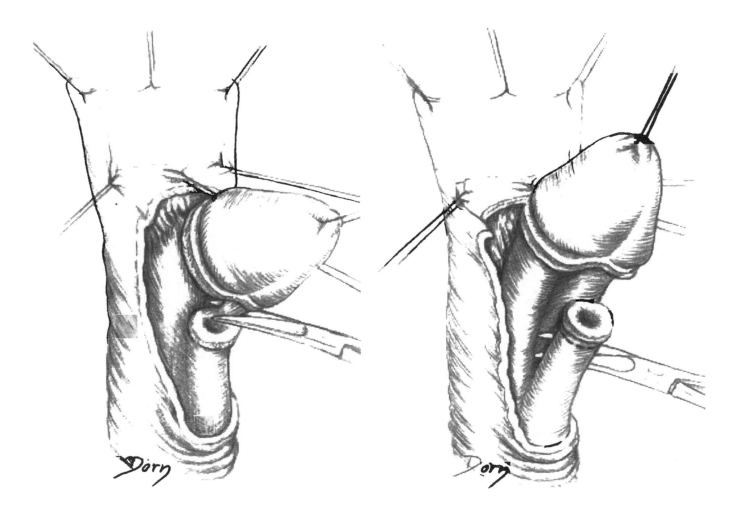

E Preparation of the urethra: excision of the meatus and the distal hypoplastic portion of the urethra; incision of the inferior aspect of the urethra and fixation of the dorsal aspect of the corpus spongiosum to the corpora cavernosa.

F The mucosal flap is isolated on its pedicle.

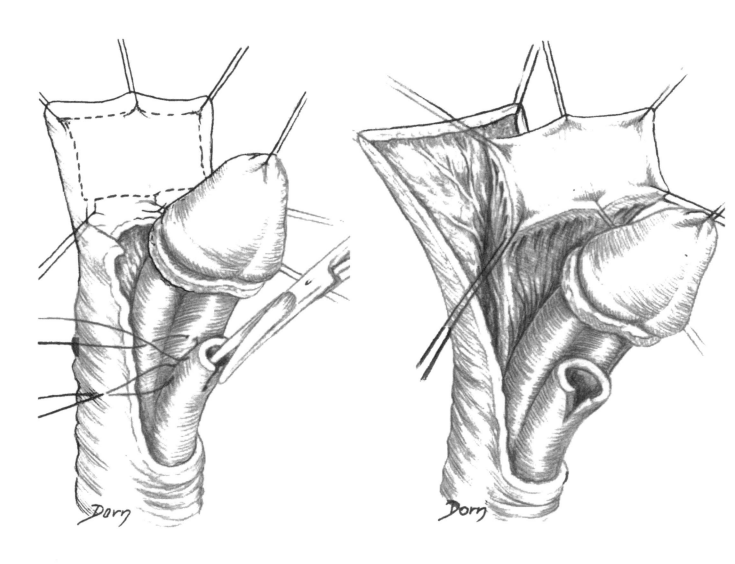

G   Tubularisation of the flap. Note the trough in the glans to implant the neo-urethra.

H   The reconstruction is covered by a skin flap.

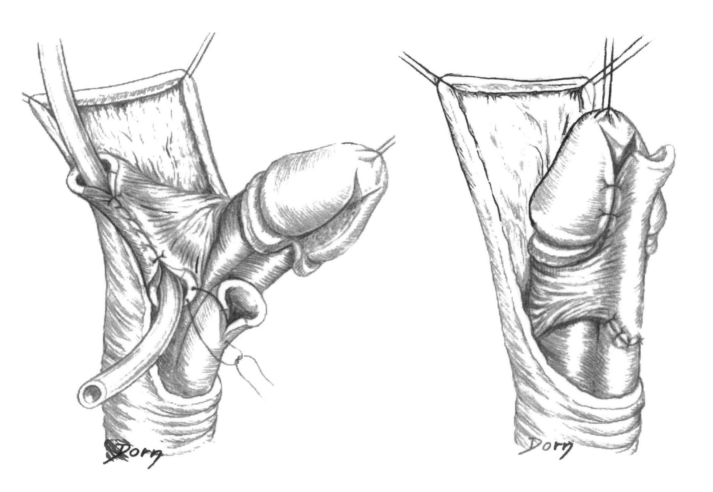

Prosthesis for erectile function of penis

The principle is to obtain an artificial erection by inflating the corpora cavernosa of the penis. The glans penis cannot be erected by this prosthesis.

A Prosthesis of penis. It comprises a tank, a pump and two inflatable cylinders which will be placed in the corpora cavernosa.

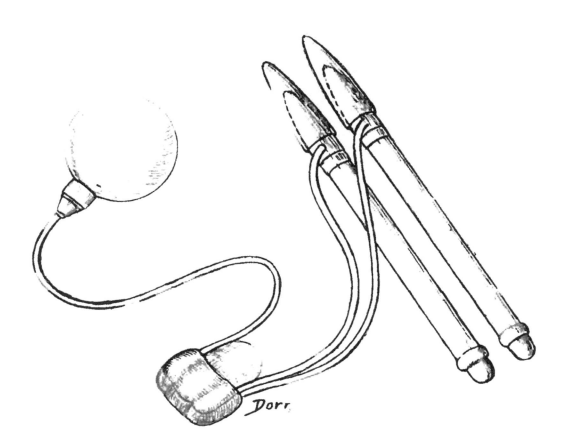

B, C The prosthesis in the flaccid state and in erection. The tank is placed in Retzius' space while the pump is in the scrotum.

B

C

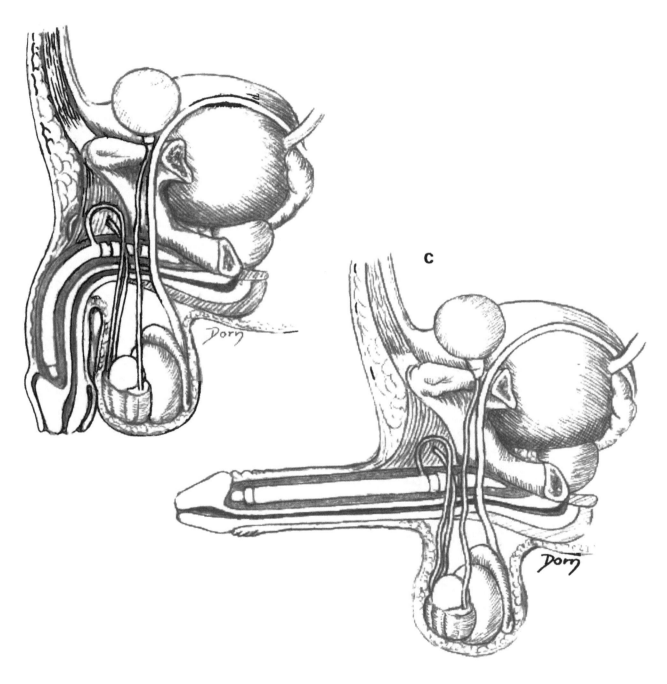

D–G Surgical procedure. Incision of the corpus cavernosum and dilation.

D

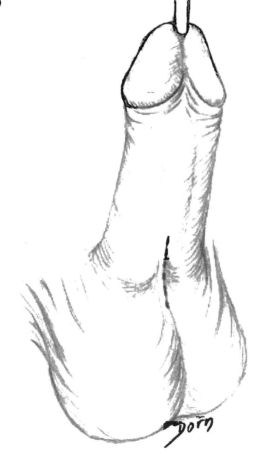

E

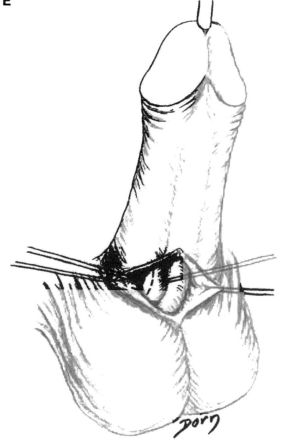

F

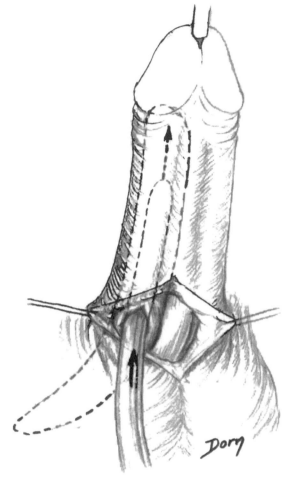

G

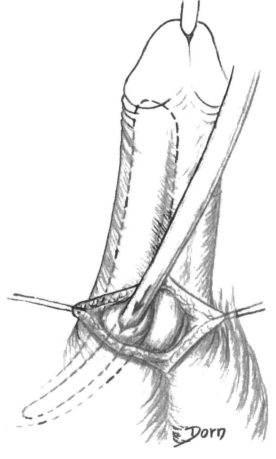

H A needle with a thread is passed through the glans, which permits lifting up the cylinder to put it in right place.

I The same procedure is performed on the other corpus cavernosum.

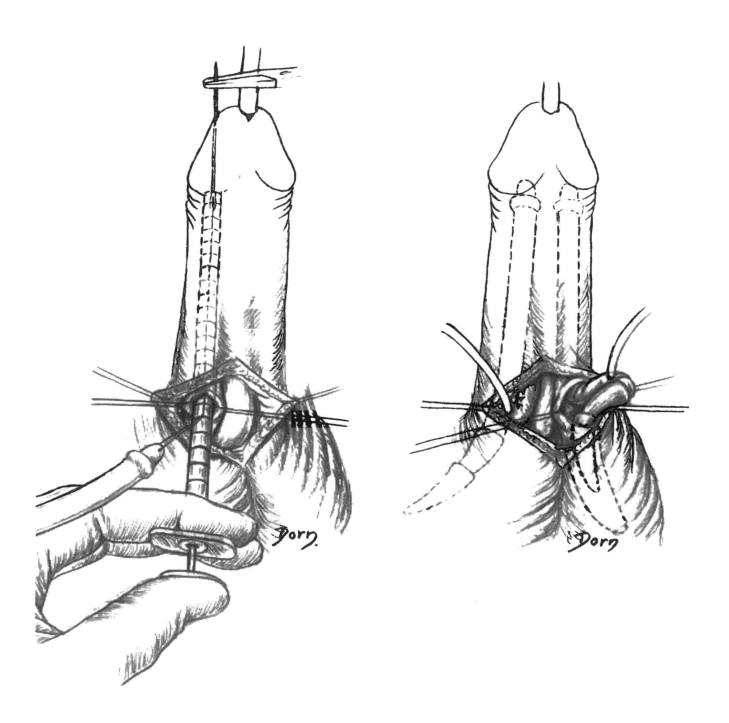

J   A tunnel is made in the scrotum to place the pump.

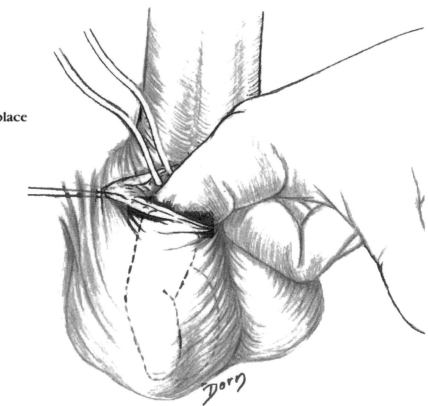

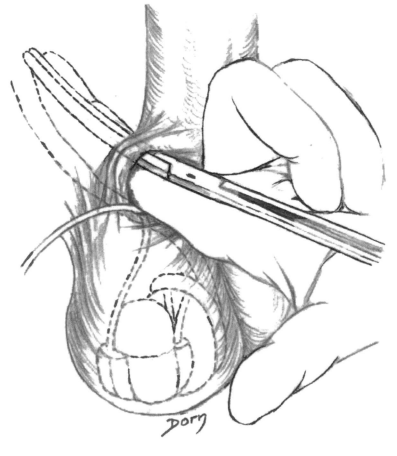

K   A tunnel is made to give access to Retzius' space (for the tank).

L   The tank is introduced with a small speculum.

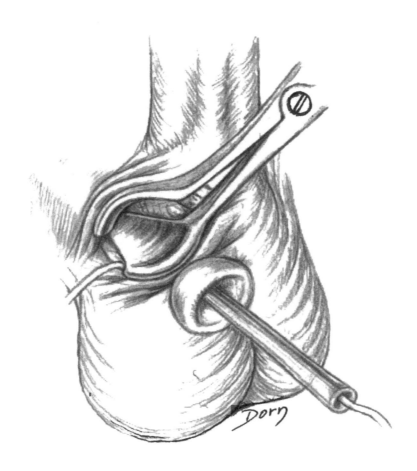

Amputation of the penis for sexual ambiguity: feminisation

A Diagrammatic representation of sexual ambiguity. Note the short urogenital sinus.

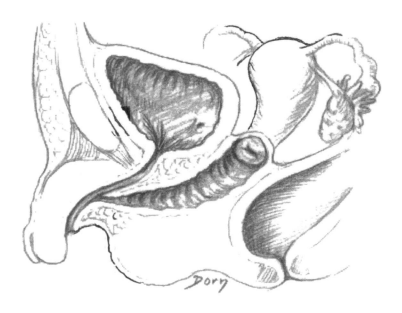

B Vagina plasty and plasty of the labia. The skin incision permits raising a large flap with a posterior hinge.

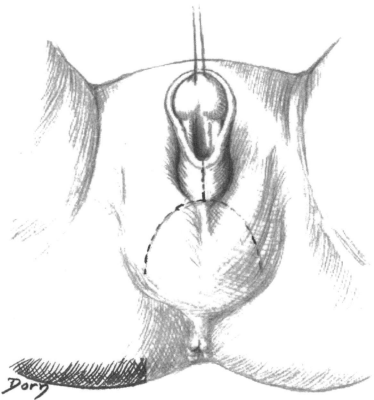

C, D Incision in the posterior aspect of the urogenital sinus.

C

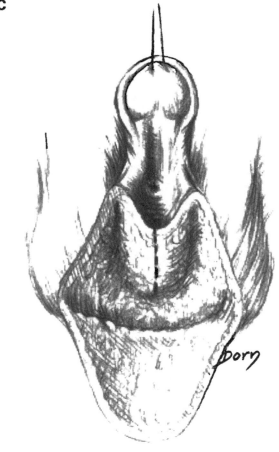

D

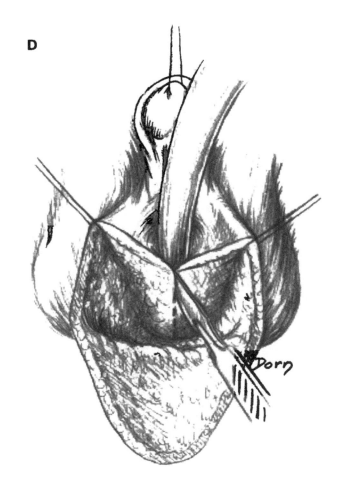

E The skin flap is inserted in the posterior aspect of the urogenital sinus (which has been incised). Incisions to prepare the plasty of the labia, the clitoris and the prepuce of the clitoris.

F Complete release of the penis; which will become the clitoris organ.

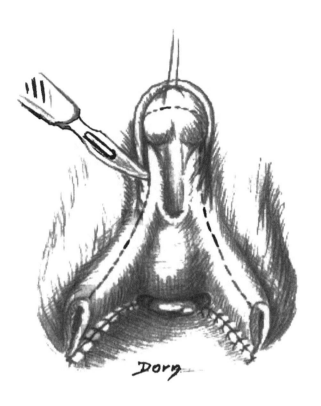

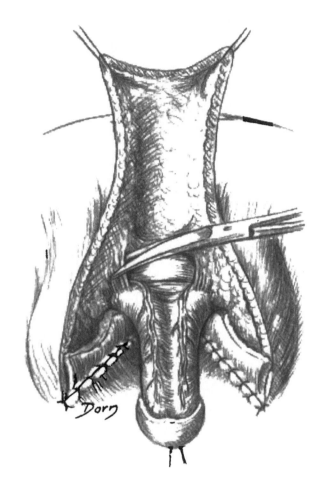

G Release of the ventral aspects of the corpora
cavernosa.

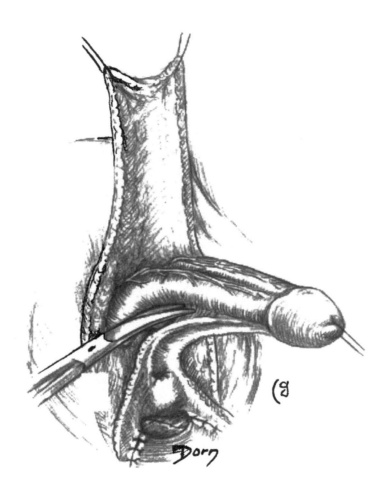

H Plasty of the clitoris. Dissection of the dorsal neurovascular pedicle for the (future) clitoris. **I** Origin of the nerves.

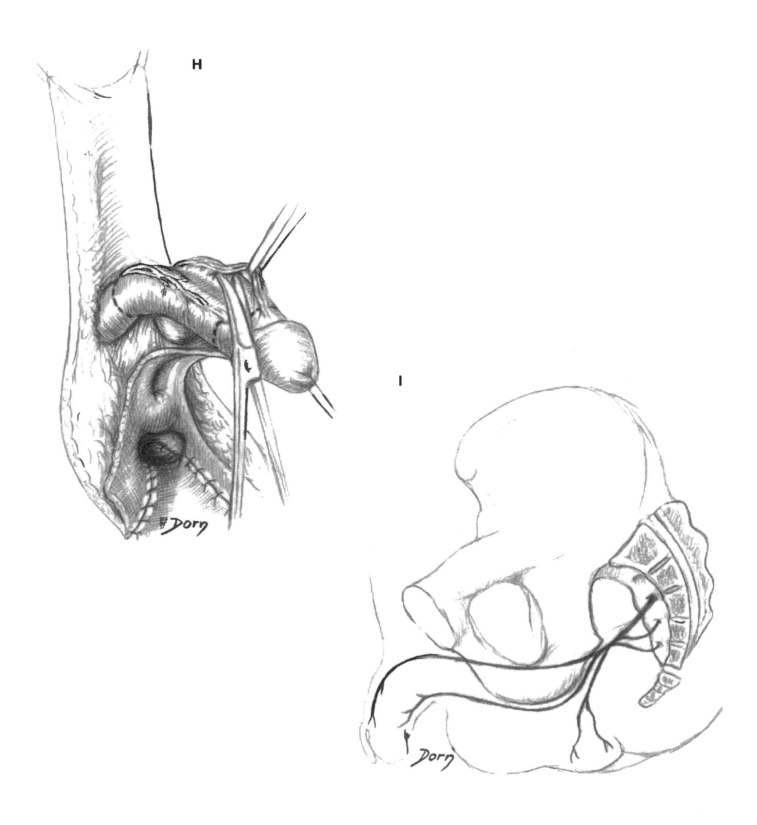

J Excision of the major portions of the corpora cavernosa, taking care of the neurovascular pedicles which supply the glans.

K Suture. The penis is shortened to obtain a clitoris.

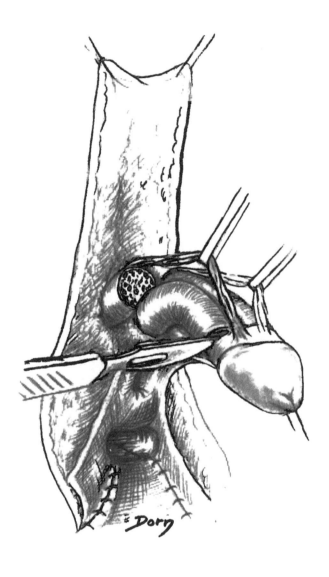

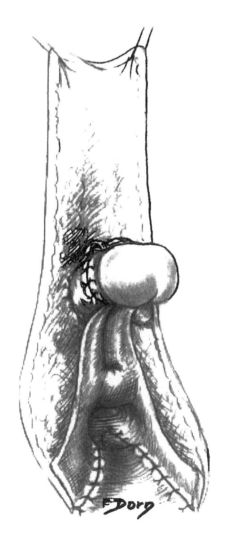

L   Plasty of the labium minus.

M   Reconstruction of the labium majus and labium minus.

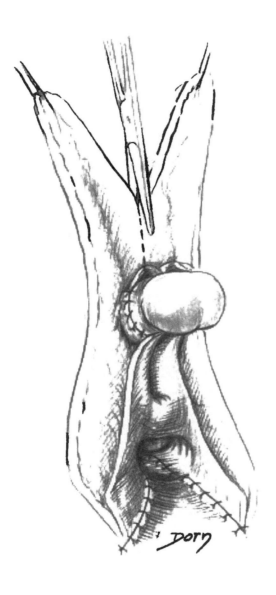

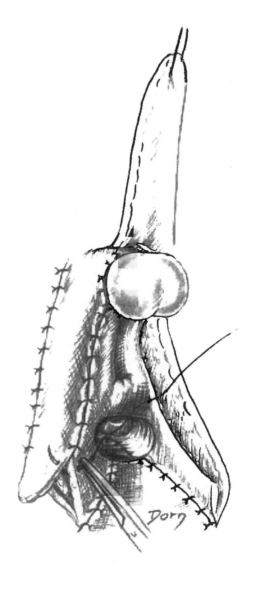

N Final aspect.

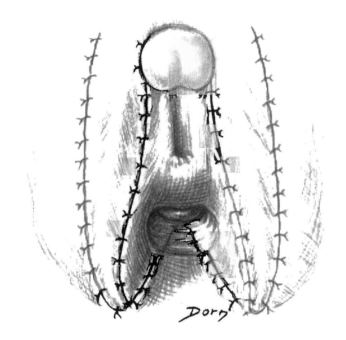

5

Abdominal surgery

The following series of illustrations is devoted to surgery of the abdominal viscera. The organs of the abdomen can be removed in case of tumour-like cancer; they can also be used in palliative procedures to reconstruct another organ which has been removed. The ileum, which is the distal portion of the small intestine, is not absolutely indispensable for normal physiology; it is routinely employed to replace a missing bladder.

Great advances have been made in liver surgery recently, particularly in the field of transplantation. The division of the liver into segments is based upon ramification of bile ducts and hepatic vessels and does not entirely correspond with division into lobes. Segmental resections are of major interest in traumatology and surgery of liver tumours. One of the main recent advances is the possibility of transferring a lobe from the liver of a living donor to replace an entire liver in a recipient patient.

Abdominal surgery

Reconstruction of a urinary bladder

A The distal portion of the ileum is isolated with the corresponding part of mesentery.

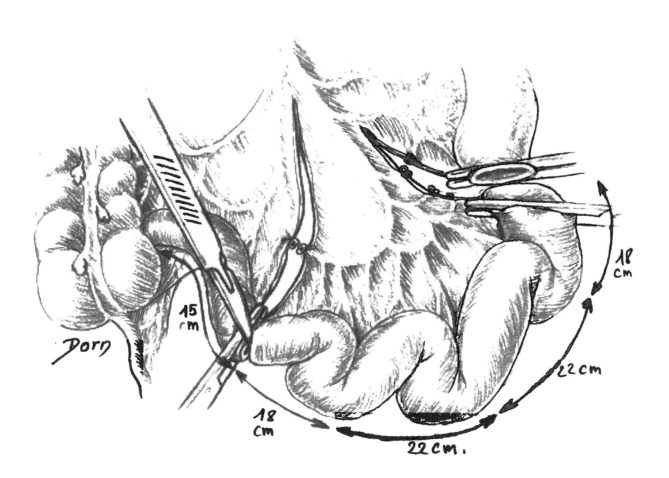

B The ileum is opened and sutured to reproduce a bladder.

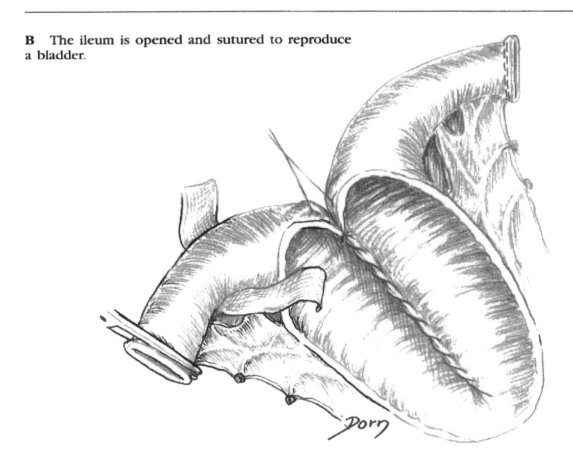

C Invagination of the afferent extremity to perform an antiretrograde flow valve.

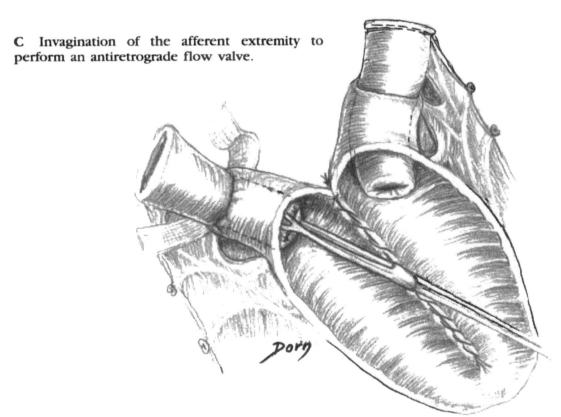

D Stabilisation of the invaginated extremity by staples.

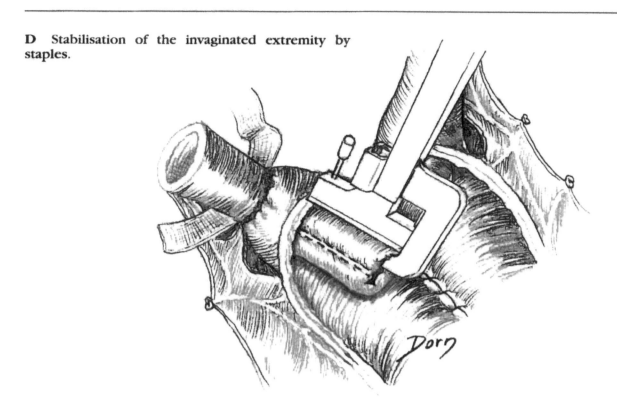

E Suture of the 'pocket'.

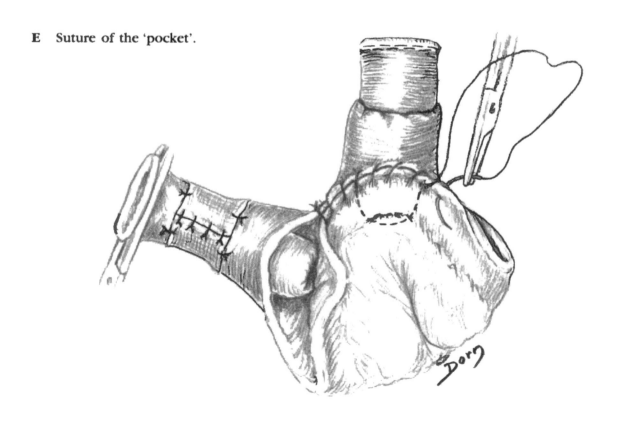

F The two ureters are implanted in the afferent
extremity. The efferent extremity is passed through
the abdominal wall to constitute a stomy.

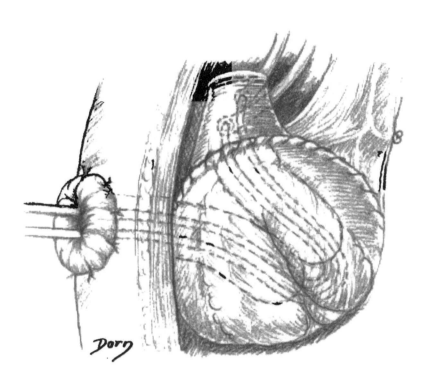

Gastrectomy

• **Oesogastrectomy for cancer.**

The tumour is located near the cardia.

A, B Excision of the proximal two-thirds of the stomach and the distal part of the oesophagus.

A

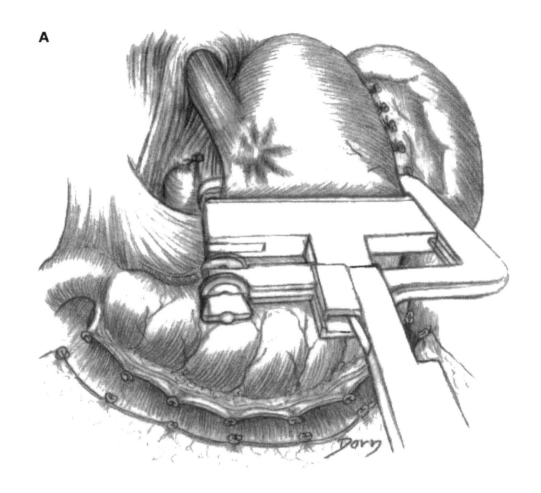

B

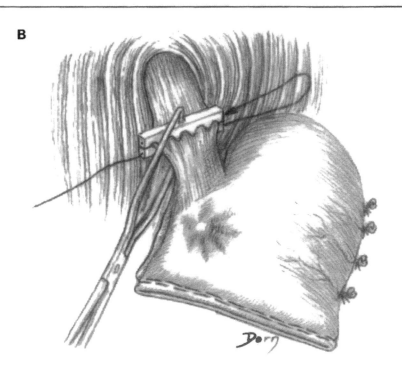

C The distal portion of the stomach is lifted up and anastomosed with the oesophagus.

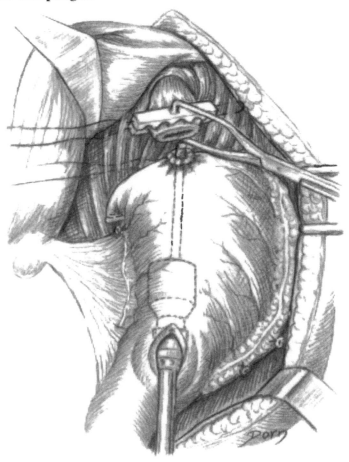

• gastrectomy and anastomoses with the jejunum.

D–F The distal two-thirds of the stomach is isolated and removed. The extremities of the remaining portion of the stomach and of the jejunum are closed with mechanical staples.

D

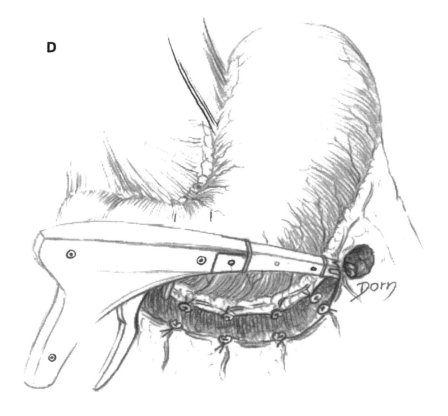

E

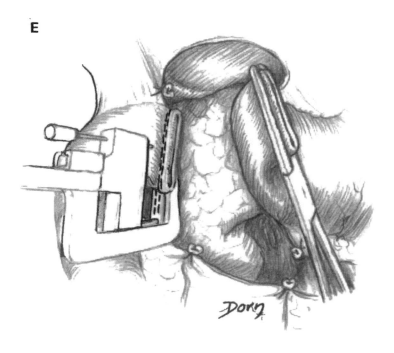

F

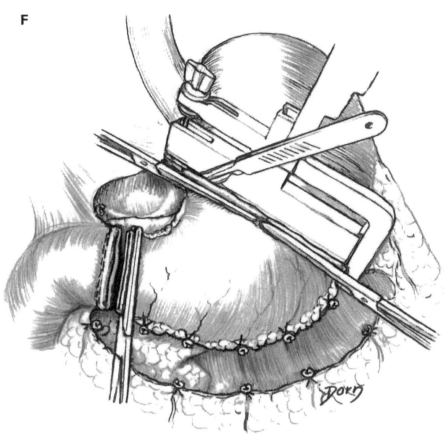

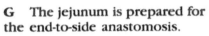

G The jejunum is prepared for the end-to-side anastomosis.

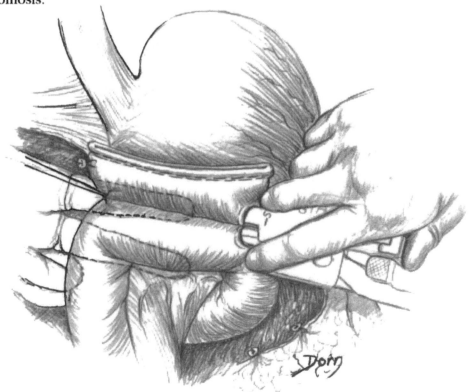

H, I Final view of the procedure.

H

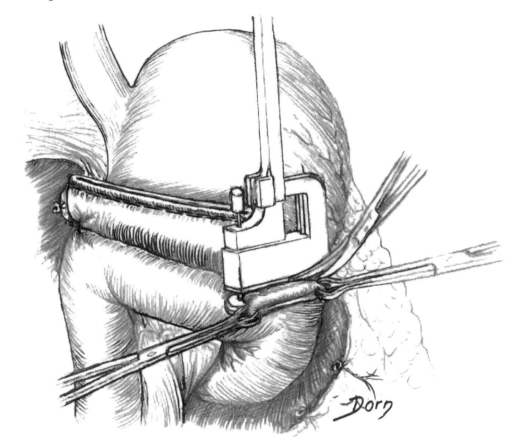

I

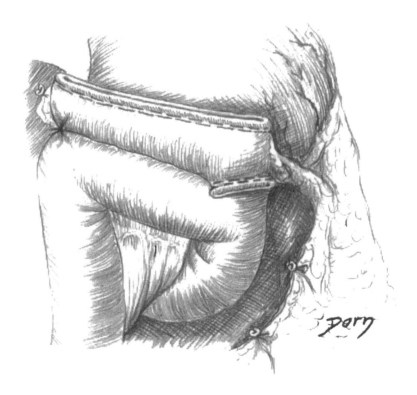

The liver

A–B The two lobes of the liver. Distribution of vessels and cuts.

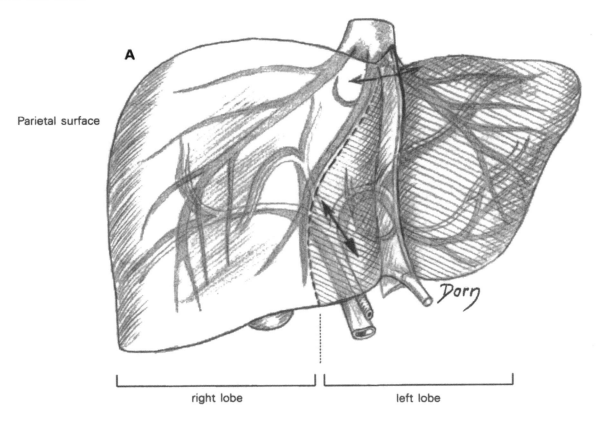

Parietal surface

right lobe | left lobe

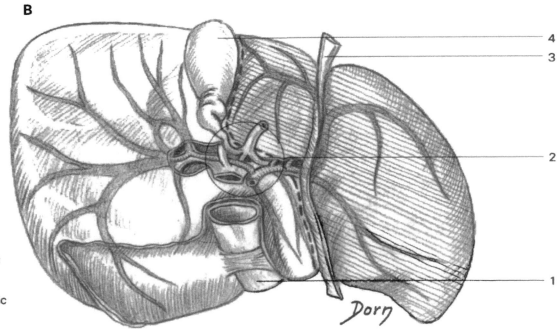

1 inferior vena cava
2 common hepatic duct, portal vein and proper hepatic artery
3 round ligament
4 gall bladder

C, D Anatomic variation of the distribution. The
left lobe is less developed.

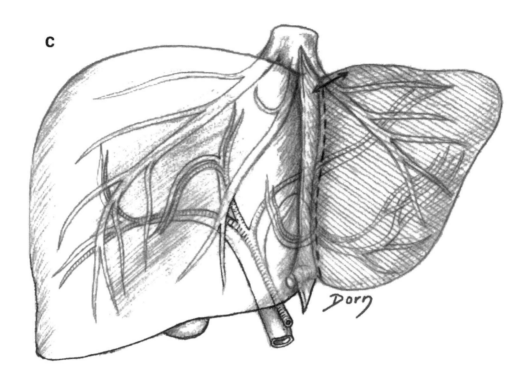

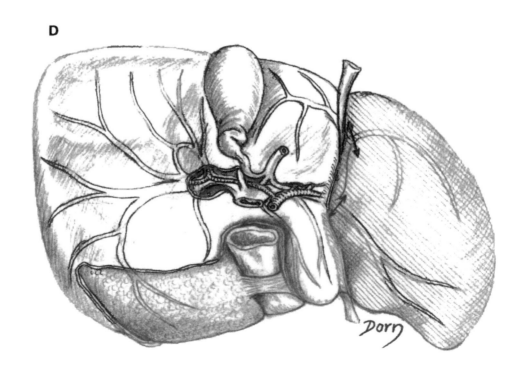

E, F Left hepatectomy.

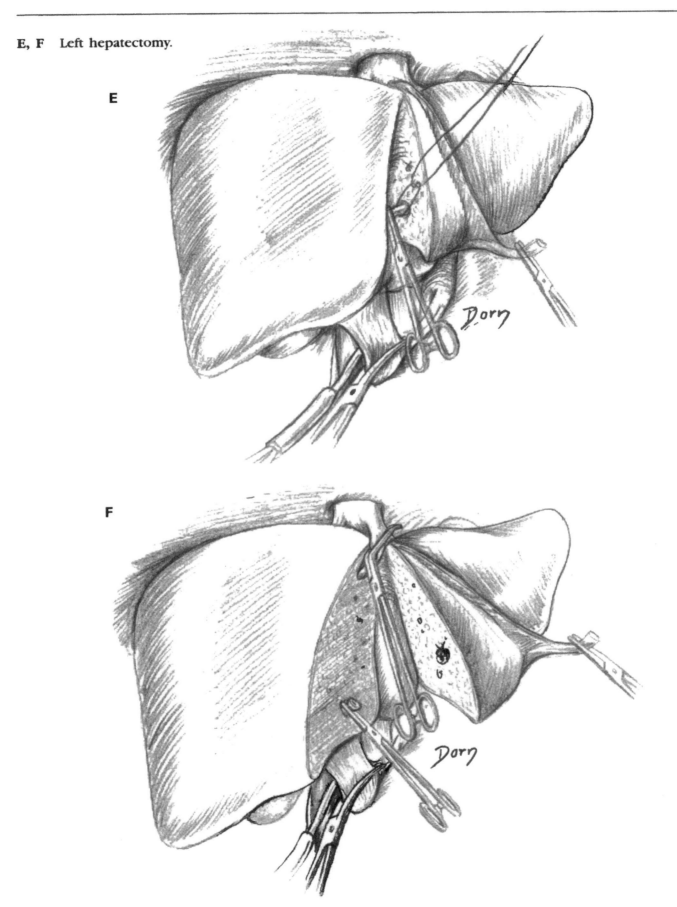

G, H   Partial left hepatectomy.

G

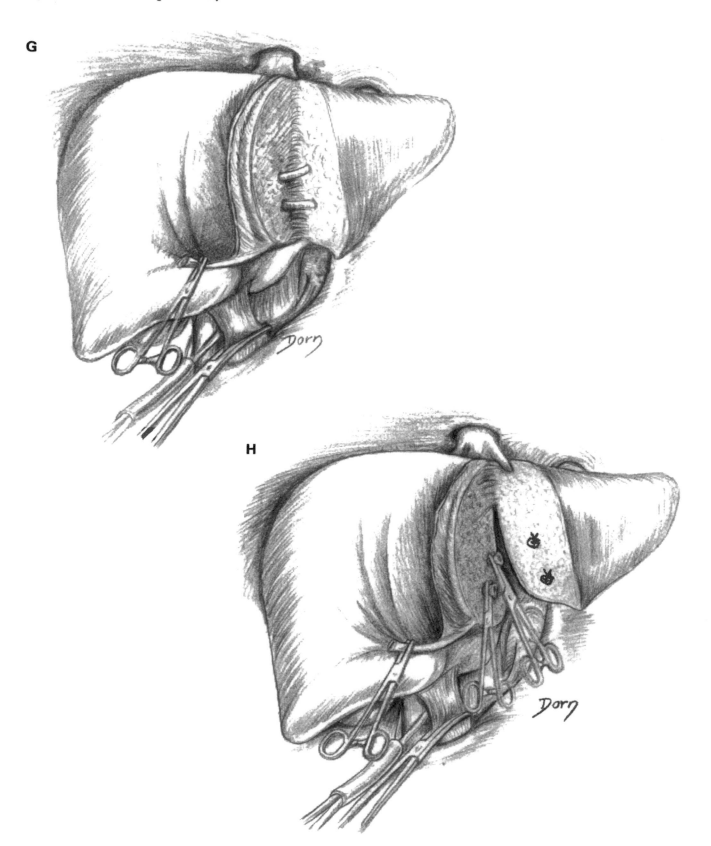

H

6

Surgery of the vertebral column

The following chapter is in a less complete or definitive fashion since the drawings were made a long time ago and many sketches were lost. However, this presentation allows us to appreciate the artistic skills of Léon Dorn, whatever the field of anatomy or surgery.

Surgery of the vertebral column

Transpleural approach to the dorsal rachis by thoracotomy

A The posterolateral incision is at the level of the sixth rib. The latissimus dorsi muscle is severed.

A

1 sixth rib
2 latissimus dorsi
3 trapezius
4 rhomboid
5 latissimus dorsi

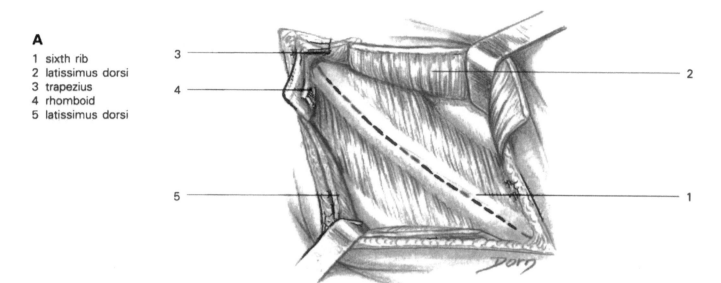

B A segment of rib has been removed. The pleura is incised.

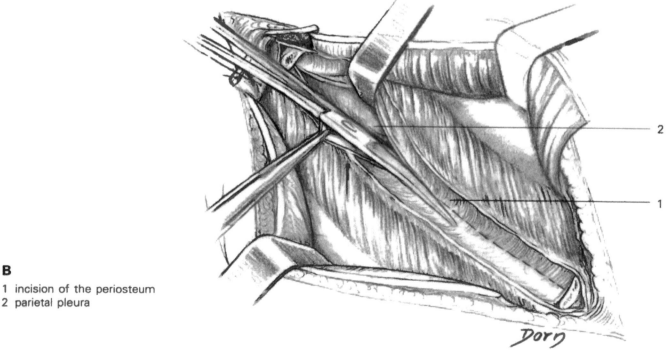

B

1 incision of the periosteum
2 parietal pleura

C Exposure of the dorsal rachis; the oesophagus, azygos vein and lung are gently retracted.

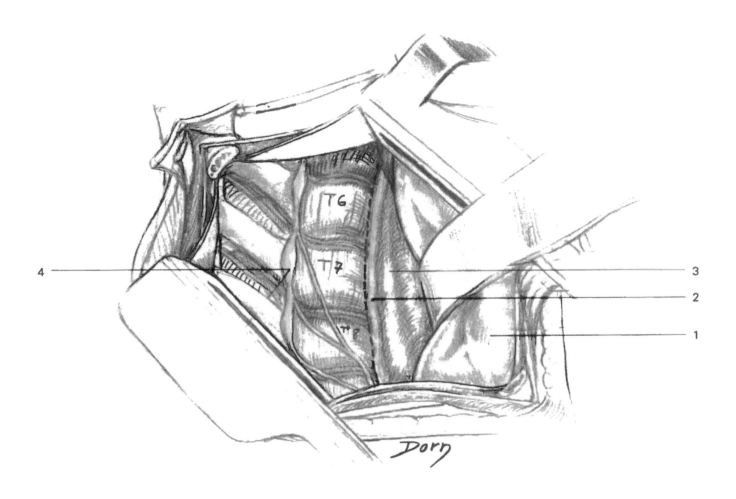

C

1 pleura and lung retracted
2 azygos vein
3 oesophagus
4 sympathetic trunk and ganglia

Surgery of the vertebral column

Treatment of lumbar spondylolisthesis

The surgical technique consists of the resection of the posterior segment of a vertebra and corporeal fusion with the underlying vertebra.

A After exposure of the affected vertebra the ligamentum flavum is excised.

B The inferior joints are opened and the capsule is excised. The superior articular facets are osteotomised.

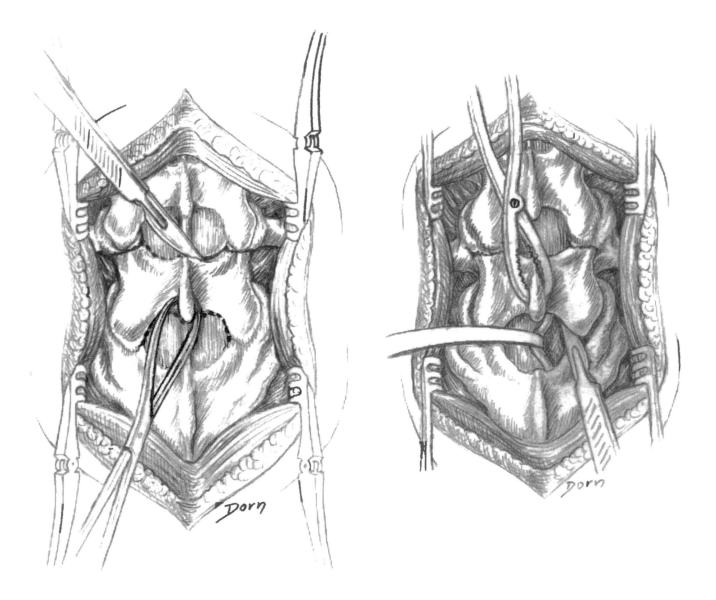

C, D The whole of the posterior portion of the vertebra is removed. The spinal cord is freed.

C

D

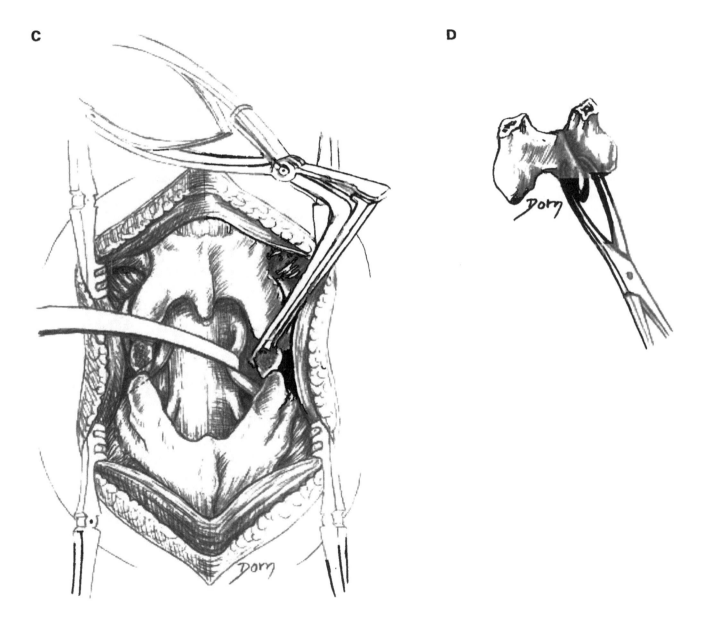

E Harvesting cancellous bone from the posterior iliac crest.

F A posterolateral fusion is prepared by putting small chips of cancellous bone on the transverse processes.

E

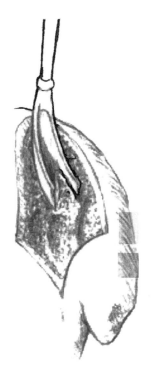

F

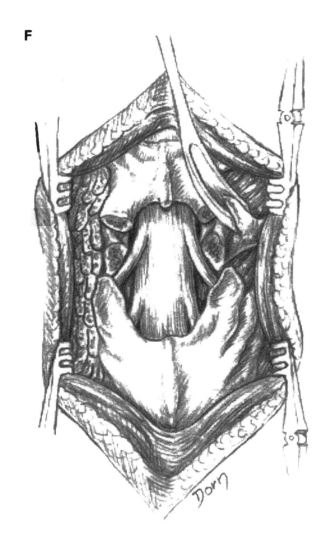

G, H   An intersomatic fusion by the same posterior approach can be combined with the posterolateral fusion or it can be performed as an alternative by the anterior approach.

G

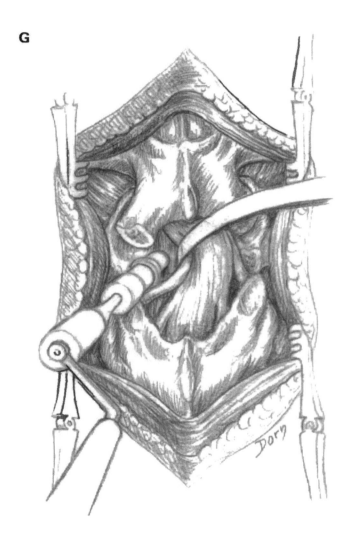

H

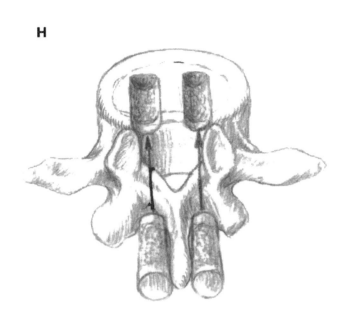

Surgical treatment of scoliosis

Different devices have been described for correction of scoliosis. This series of illustrations presents Harrington's rod, which is now considered obsolete.

A The principle of Harrington's procedure. The rod is used in distraction to correct the curvature; the extremities of the rod are fixed by hooks which are applied on the laminae of the vertebrae.

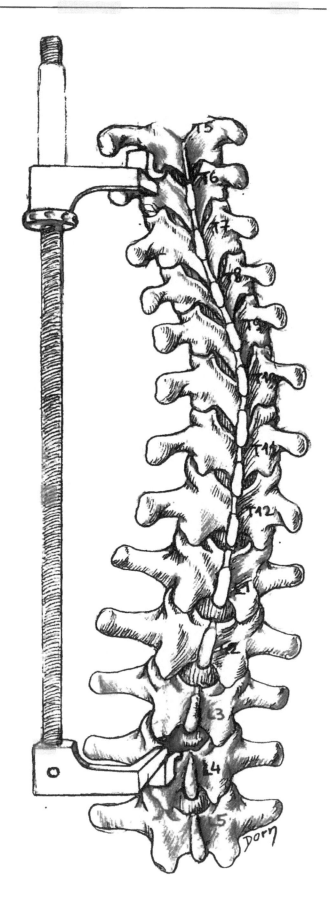

B   Small bone chips of the posterior segments of the vertebrae are removed to prepare the posterior fusion.

C, D   The inferior hook is put in place; partial bone resection is needed.

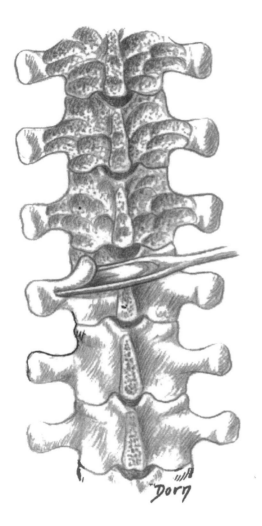

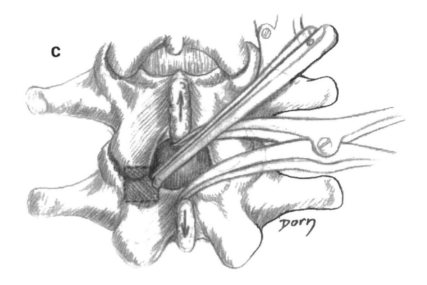

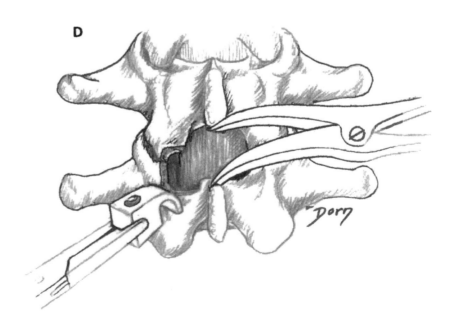

E Setting Harrington's rod and distraction to correct the curvature.

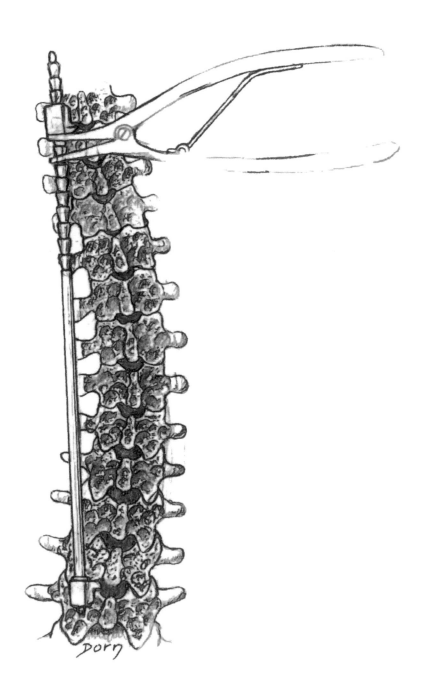

Treatment of lumbar disc hernia: anterior approach

The anterior approach to remove a disc hernia at the lumbosacral level is usually not used. It is only indicated when an intersomatic fusion is performed in the same operation; the risk is a lesion of the superior hypogastric plexus.

A A transperitoneal approach is made. The organs are retracted. The sacral promontory is exposed and the posterior peritoneum is incised.

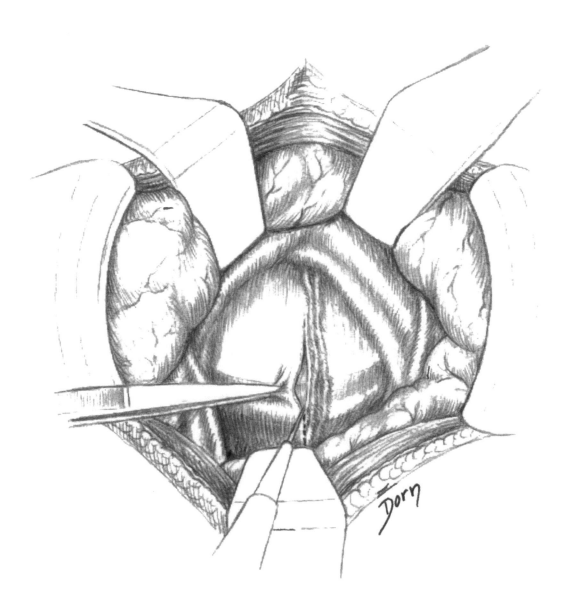

B, C The disc is exposed and the anterior longitudinal ligament is opened.

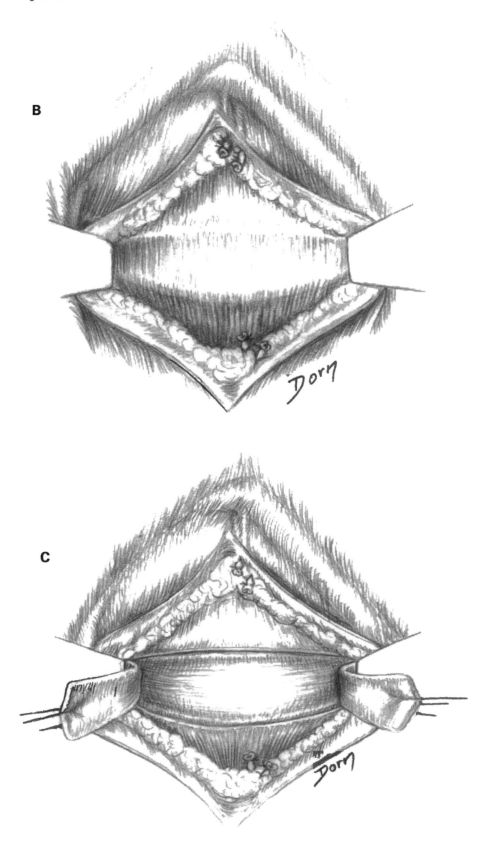

D   Excision of the disc.

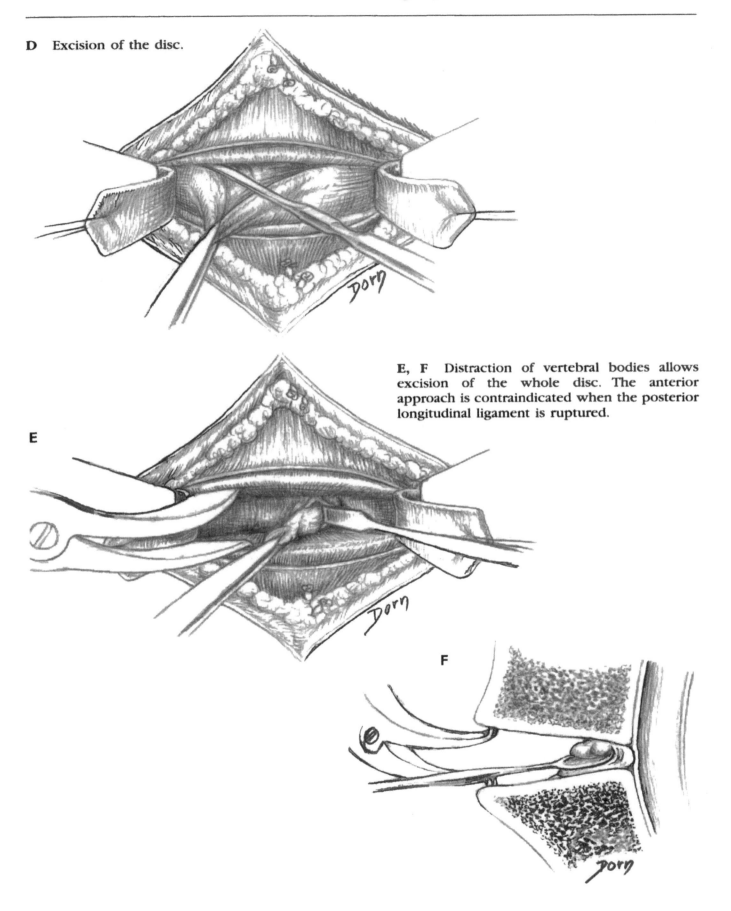

E, F   Distraction of vertebral bodies allows excision of the whole disc. The anterior approach is contraindicated when the posterior longitudinal ligament is ruptured.

E

F

7

Upper limb surgery

Surgery of the upper limb has increasingly gained interest over the past 20 years. This is due to the major development of the surgery of the hand, which is equally performed by orthopaedic and plastic surgeons. Moreover many recent advances have been made in the field of surgery of the shoulder and elbow, chiefly in relation to the possibilities offered by arthroscopy and prosthetic replacements. Thus, we have given some examples of surgery of the upper limb in a separate section instead of including them in the chapter on surgery of the hand and wrist.

Sternoclavicular dislocation

A Skin incision.

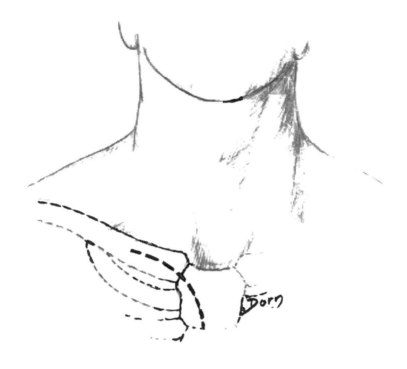

B The exposure of the sternoclavicular joint. Note the rupture of the costoclavicular ligament.

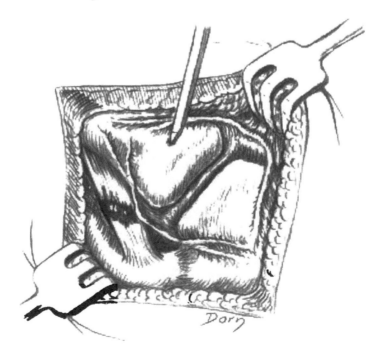

C, D Repair of the costoclavicular ligament and stabilisation by a frame or a screw.

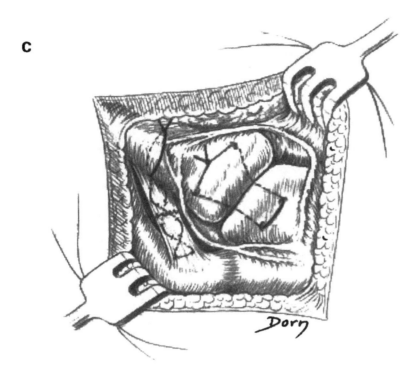

C

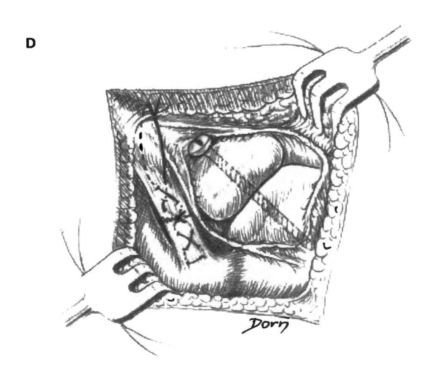

D

Stabilisation of a shoulder prosthetic implant

This type of implant is employed in comminutive fractures of the proximal extremity of the humerus.

A, B The prosthesis is put in place. The greater and the lesser tubercles are reduced on the prosthesis and firmly fixed.

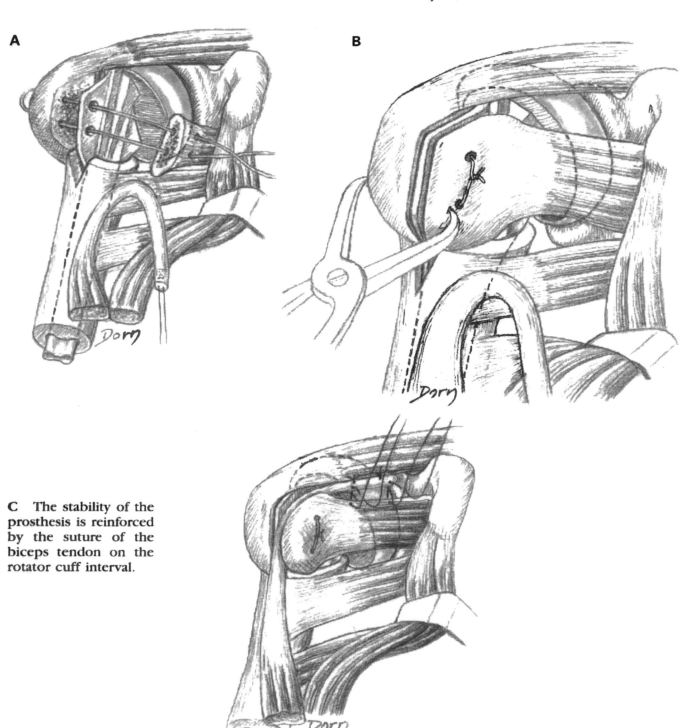

A

B

C The stability of the prosthesis is reinforced by the suture of the biceps tendon on the rotator cuff interval.

Cleidectomy

Excision of the clavicle is an uncommon procedure.
It can be indicated in case of tumour.

A   It is easier to remove the clavicle in two parts
and the procedure begins by severing the clavicle.
First all the muscle insertions are released.

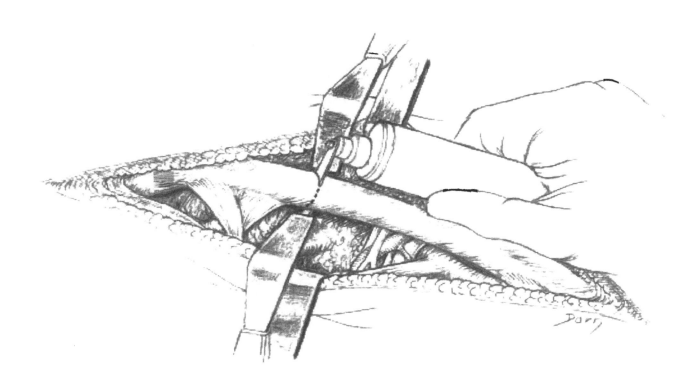

B Then the medial portion is removed by cutting the costoclavicular ligament and opening the sterno-clavicular joint.

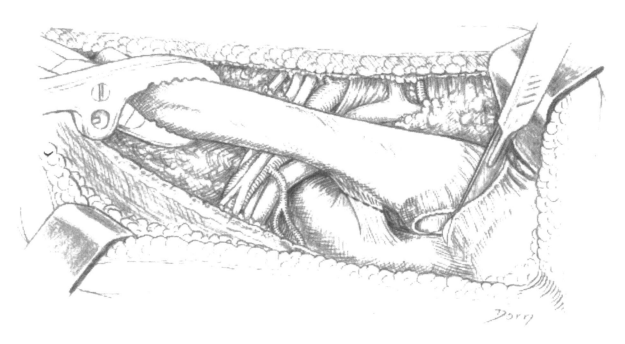

C The lateral part is removed by cutting the coracoclavicular ligament and opening the acromio-clavicular joint.

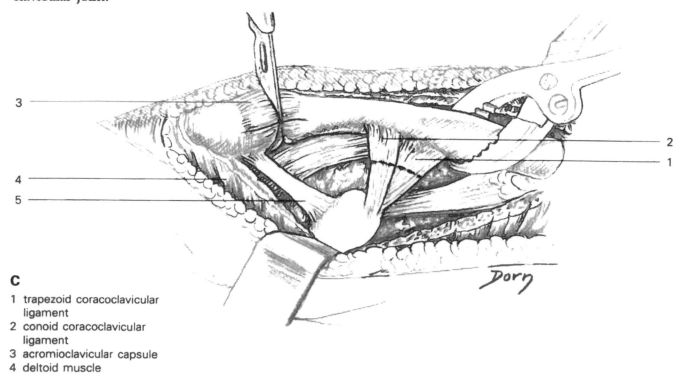

C

1 trapezoid coracoclavicular ligament
2 conoid coracoclavicular ligament
3 acromioclavicular capsule
4 deltoid muscle
5 coracoacromial ligament

Osteosynthesis of a fracture of the forearm

The following early series of drawings allows us to assess the evolution of Dorn's style. As a matter of fact, this technique was designed in 1970 for Merle d'Aubigné. Very few details are visible in the soft tissues and the shape of the bones is approximate.

A Fracture of the radius treated by a plate.

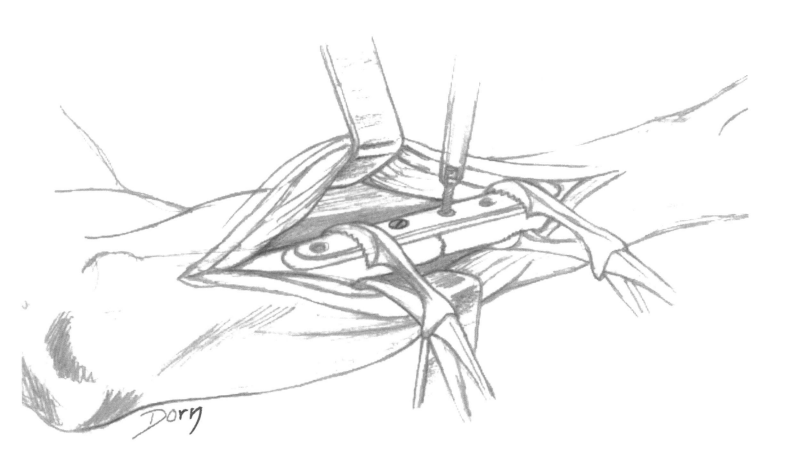

B, C The shaft of the ulna is reamed to put an intramedullar nail. The technique with exposure of the fracture site is obsolete.

B

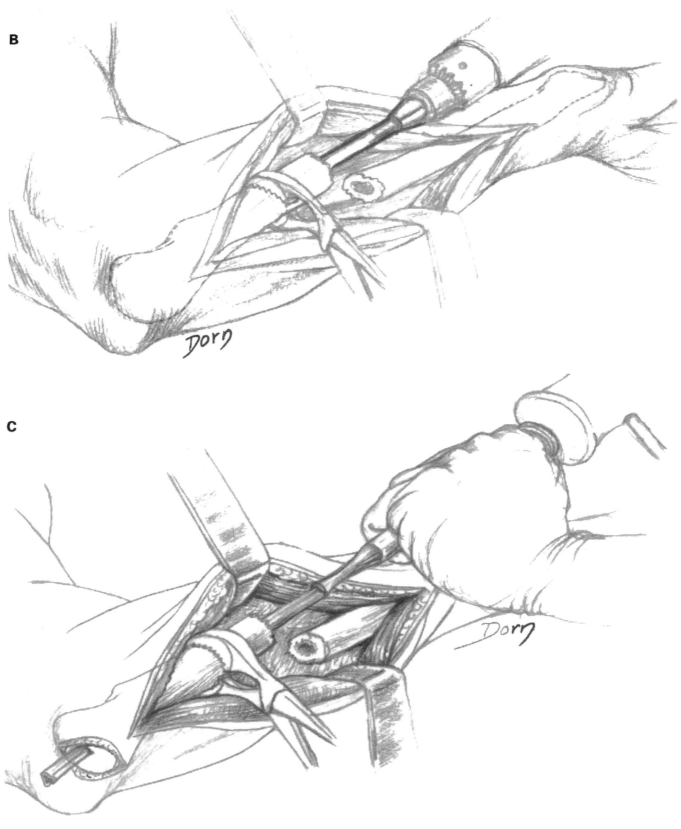

C

Surgical exposure of the shoulder

Anterior approach to the subacromial space

A Skin incision according to the bony landmarks.

B, C The deltoid origin is raised from the acromion and lateral clavicle.

B

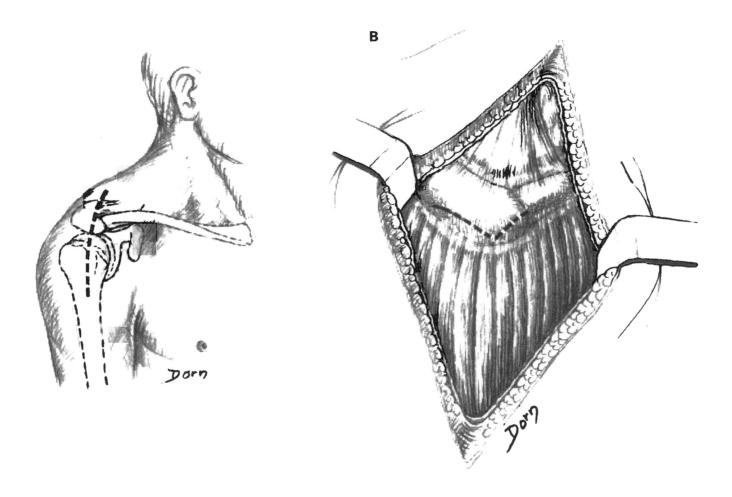

D   Exposure and incision of the subdeltoid bursa.

C

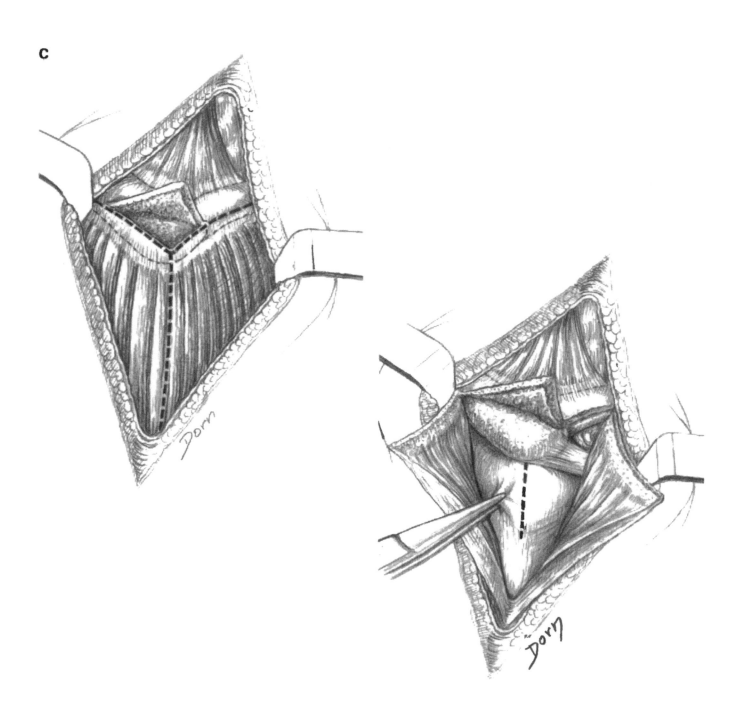

E Musculoperiosteal flaps are reinserted by fixation to the bone.

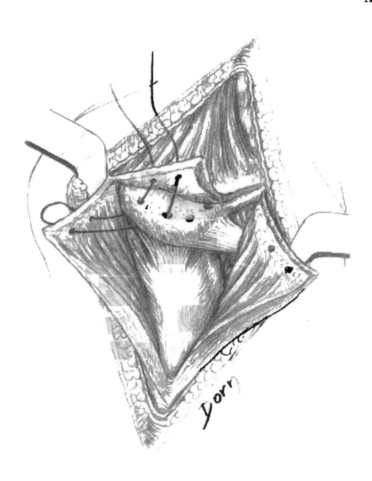

Anterior approach to the glenohumeral joint

A Skin incision.

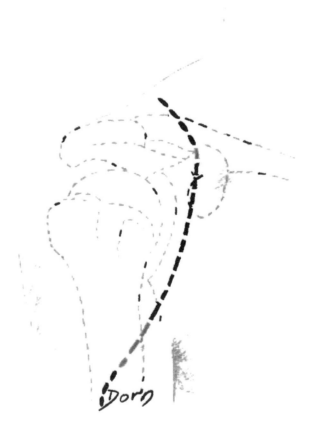

B The deltopectoral groove is opened.

C Exposure of the coracobiceps by retracting the deltoid and the pectoralis major muscles.

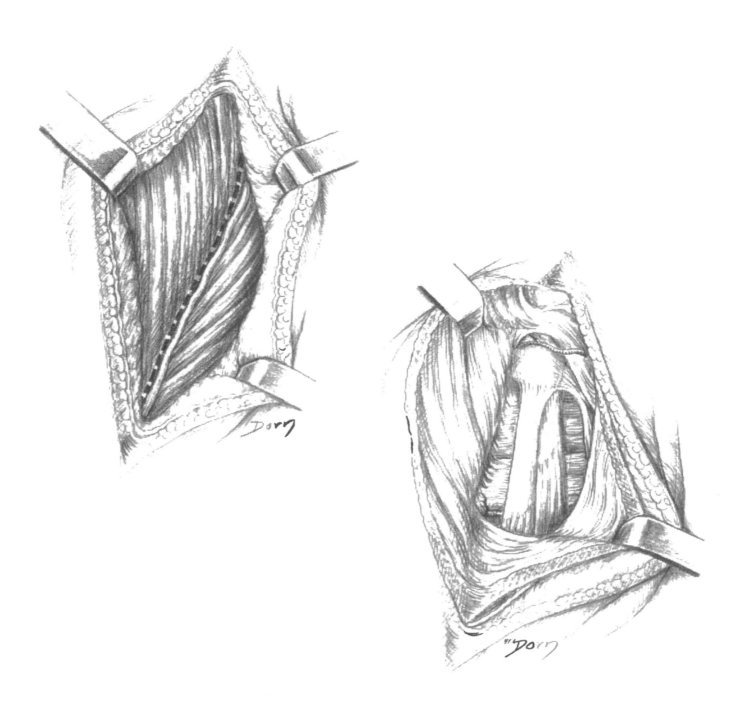

D, E The tip of the coracoid process is osteo-tomised. The coracobiceps is retracted, exposing the subscapularis muscle.

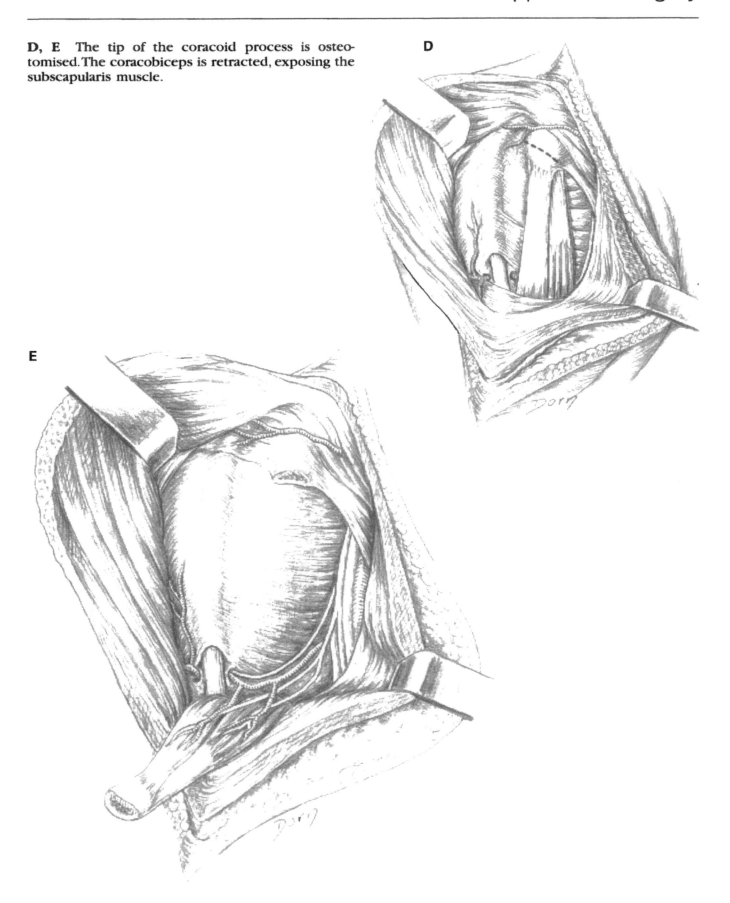

F   The tendon of the subscapularis is severed and retracted. Exposure of the capsule.

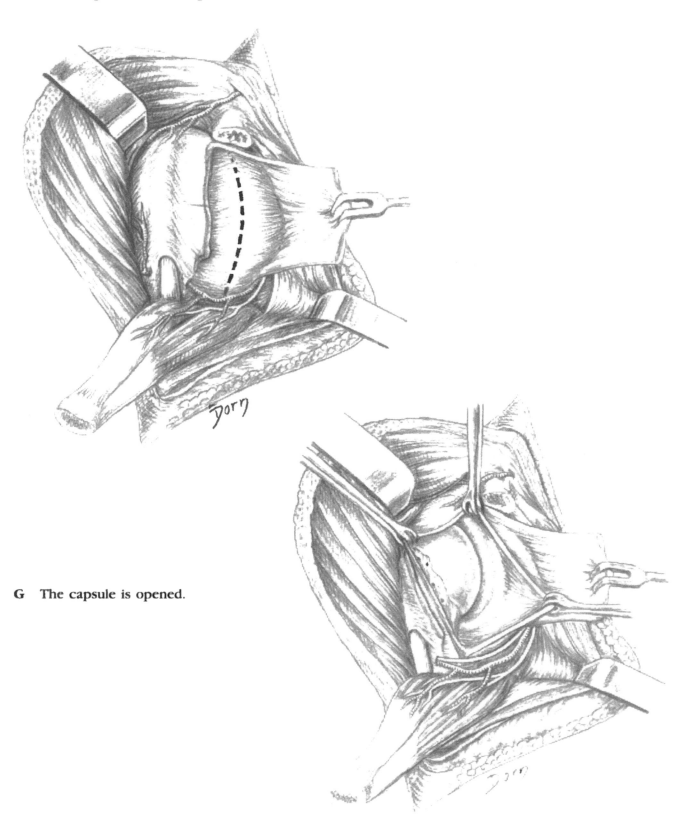

G   The capsule is opened.

Axillary approach to the glenohumeral joint

Although rarely used because of the dissection of the neurovascular pedicles, this approach has the main advantage of a cosmetically acceptable scar.

A Skin incision.

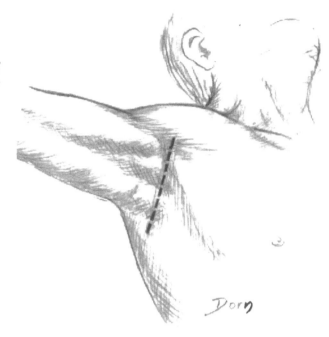

B The neurovascular bundle is lying in the axillary fat.

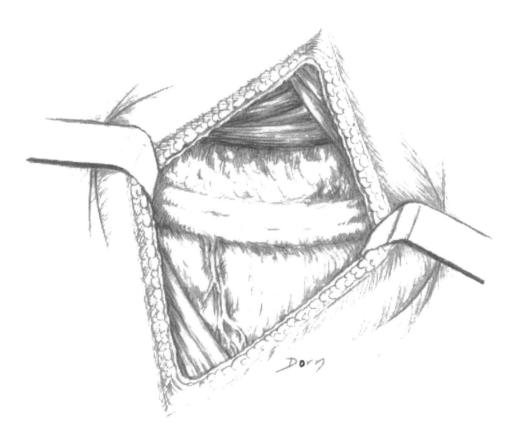

C The cords of the plexus and the vessels are visible.

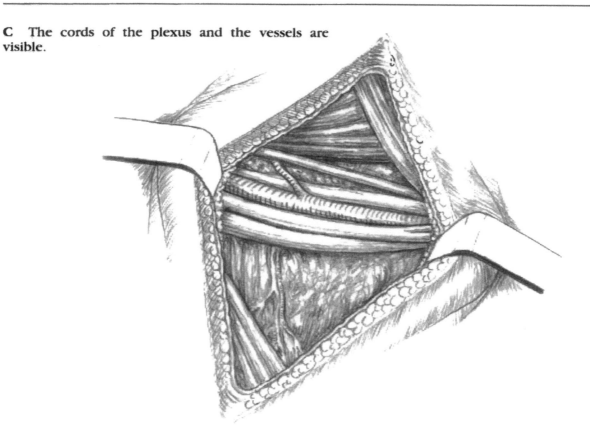

D Approach to the joint between the axillary nerve and the other components of the neurovascular bundle.

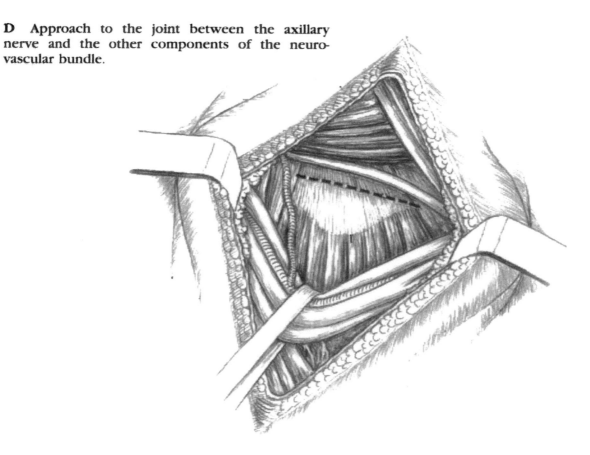

E The subscapularis tendon is served and retracted.

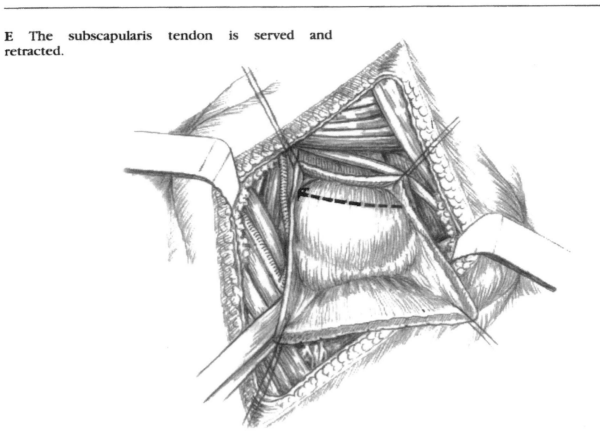

F Exposure of the joint.

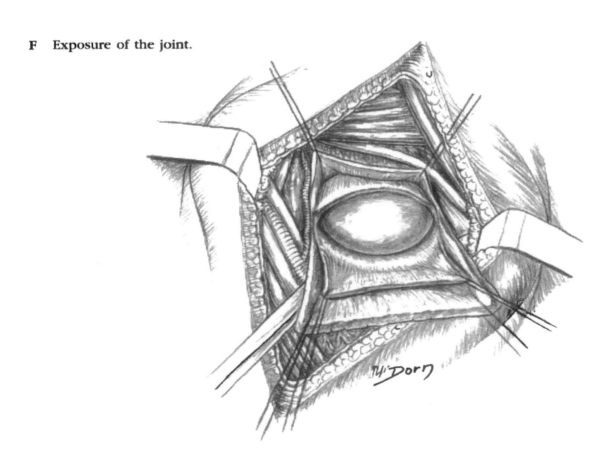

Subdeltoid approach to the proximal metaphysis of the humerus

This approach is rarely used. Its indications are tumours and malunited fractures.

A The skin incision has a U shape.

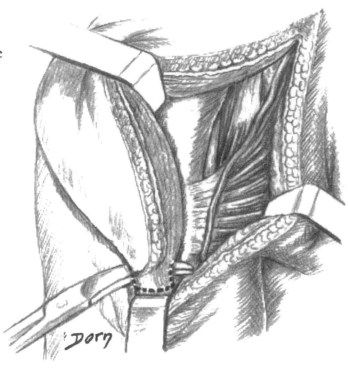

B The distal insertion of the deltoid is released with a bone block. the skin flap and the deltoid are retracted *en bloc*.

1 axillary nerve

Anterior approach to the proximal third of the radius

A The approach is made with the forearm in supination. the brachioradialis muscle is retracted laterally exposing the two branches of the radial nerve and the supinator muscle. The biceps are retracted medially. The incision is made medially to the supinator and laterally to the biceps tendon.

B Exposure of the humeroradial joint and the proximal third of the radius.

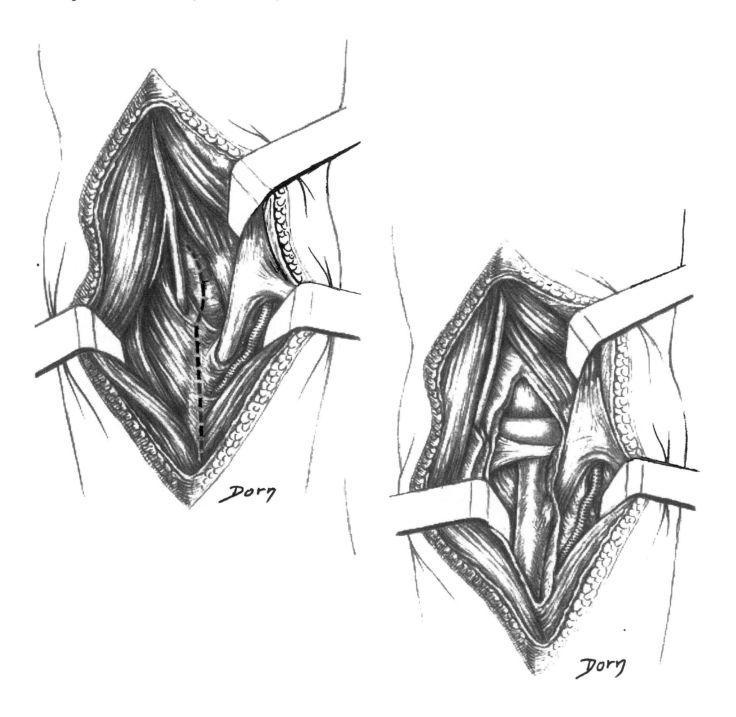

8

Lower limb surgery

The lower extremity is traditionally an important part of orthopaedic surgery; however, it is also relevant to vascular surgeons. We will survey the following: anatomy, reconstructive surgery of the knee and some approaches to the hip and the foot.

Anatomy

Anatomy of the posterior approach to
the femoral shaft

A Skin incision.

B Identification of the posterior femoral
cutaneous nerve.

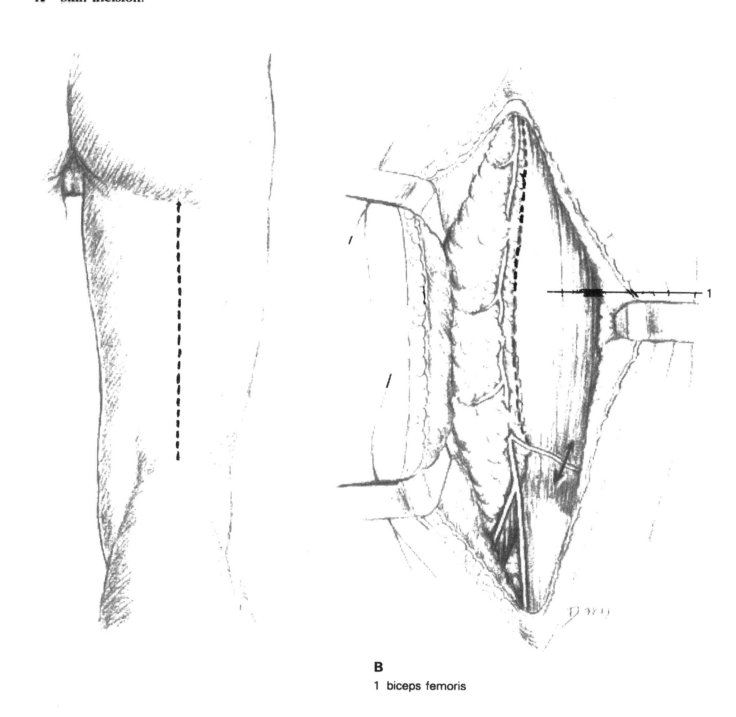

B
1 biceps femoris

C Approach between biceps and vastus lateralis. The lower part of the biceps is released from the semitendinosus.

D The long head of biceps femoris is retracted medially; the plane between the short head and vastus lateralis is developed.

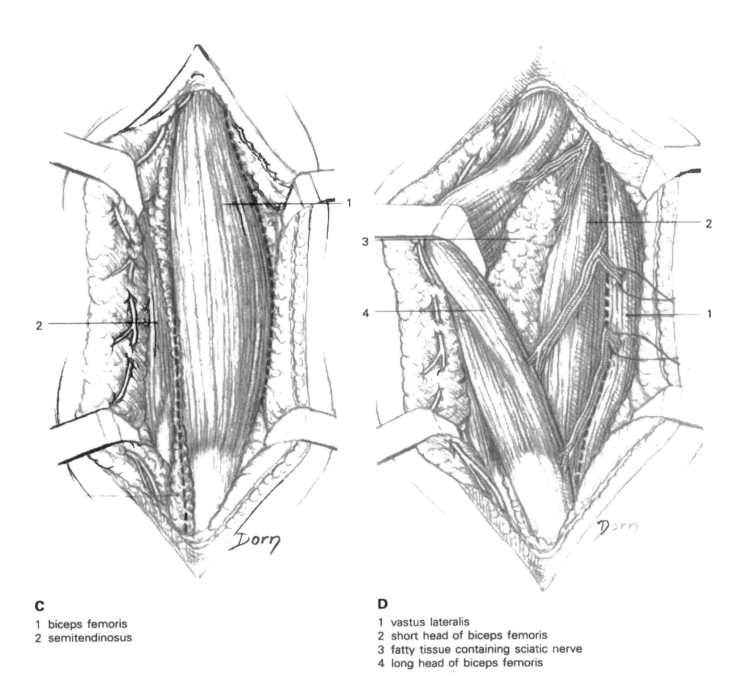

C
1 biceps femoris
2 semitendinosus

D
1 vastus lateralis
2 short head of biceps femoris
3 fatty tissue containing sciatic nerve
4 long head of biceps femoris

E Exposure of the femoral shaft.

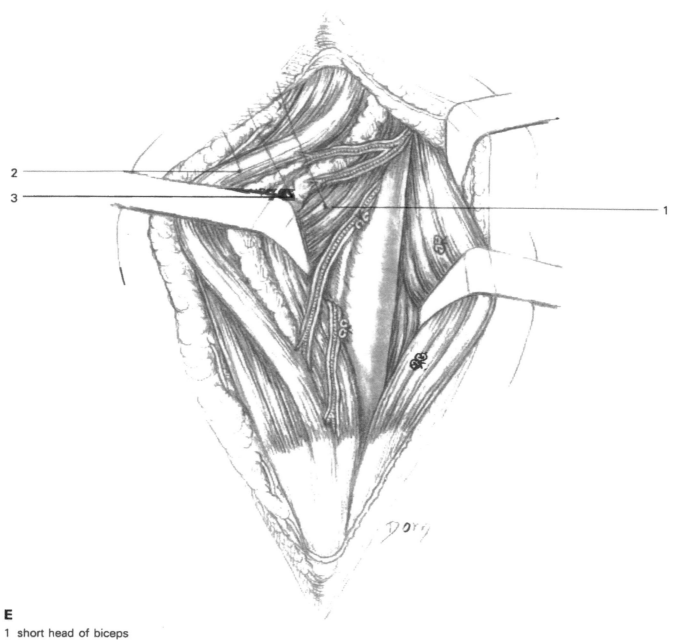

E
1 short head of biceps
2 long head of biceps
3 fatty tissue containing sciatic nerve

Extended medial approach to the popliteal vessels

A The soleus has been released from the tibia. The insertion of pes anserinus, semimembranosus and medial head of gastrocnemius are divided.

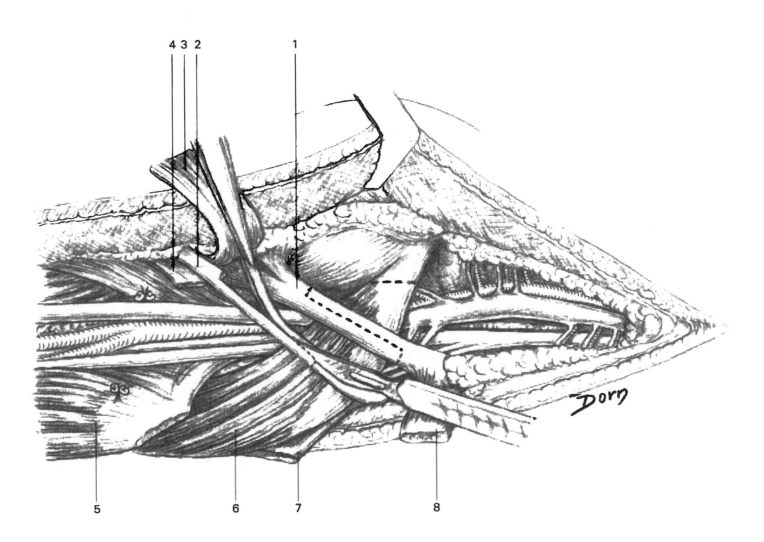

A

1 semimembranous
2 gracilis
3 sartorius
4 semitendinosus
5 soleus
6 gastrocnemius
7 semitendinosus
8 sartorius

B Medial aspect of the popliteal neurovascular bundle.

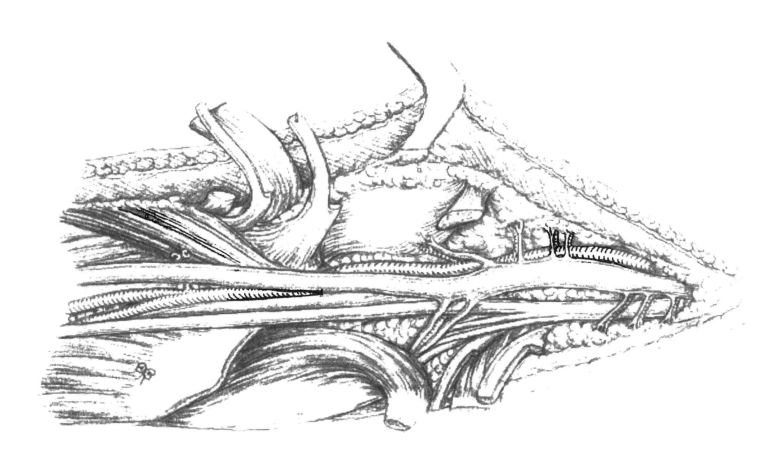

C Extended anatomical view of the medial aspect
of the knee with the vascular and nerve supply. Only
muscle insertions or tendons have been divided.

C
 1 soleus
 2 gastrocnemius
 3 sartorius
 4 gracilis
 5 semimembranosus
 6 saphenous nerve
 7 perforatory nerve
 8 adductor magnus
 9 sciatic nerve
10 femoral artery
11 vastus medialis

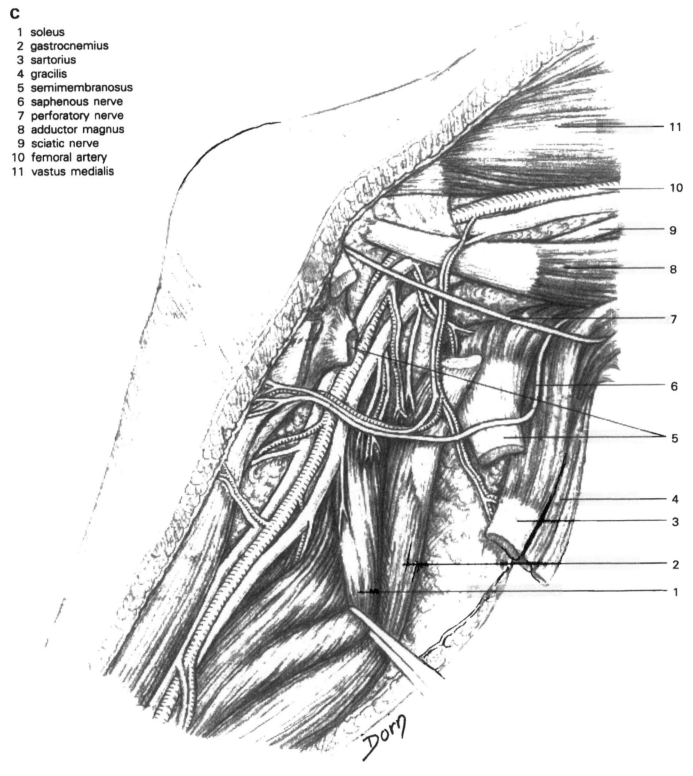

Lower limb surgery

Anatomy of the knee

A Anterior view.

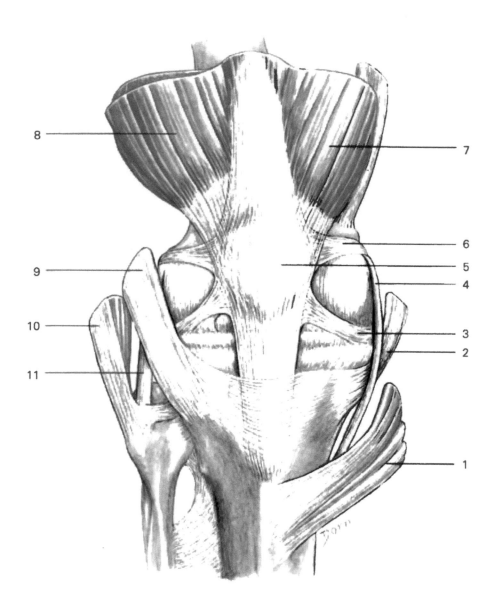

1 pes anserinus muscles
2 semimembranosus
3 patellomeniscal ligament
4 medial collateral ligament
5 patella
6 patellofemoral ligament
7 vastus medialis
8 vastus lateralis
9 iliotibial band
10 biceps femoris
11 lateral collateral ligament

B Posterior view.

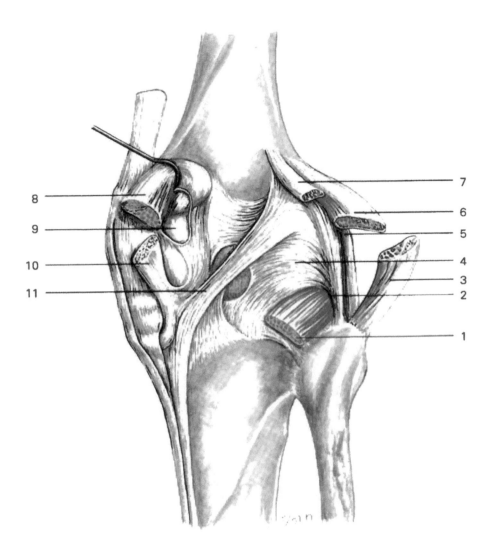

7
6
5
4
3
2
1
8
9
10
11

1 popliteus
2 popliteus hiatus
3 biceps femoris
4 arcuate ligament
5 lateral collateral ligament
6 lateral head of gastrocnemius
7 plantaris
8 medial head of gastrocnemius
9 bursa
10 semimembranosus
11 oblique ligament

Anatomy of the lumbosacral plexus

This is a definitive drawing.

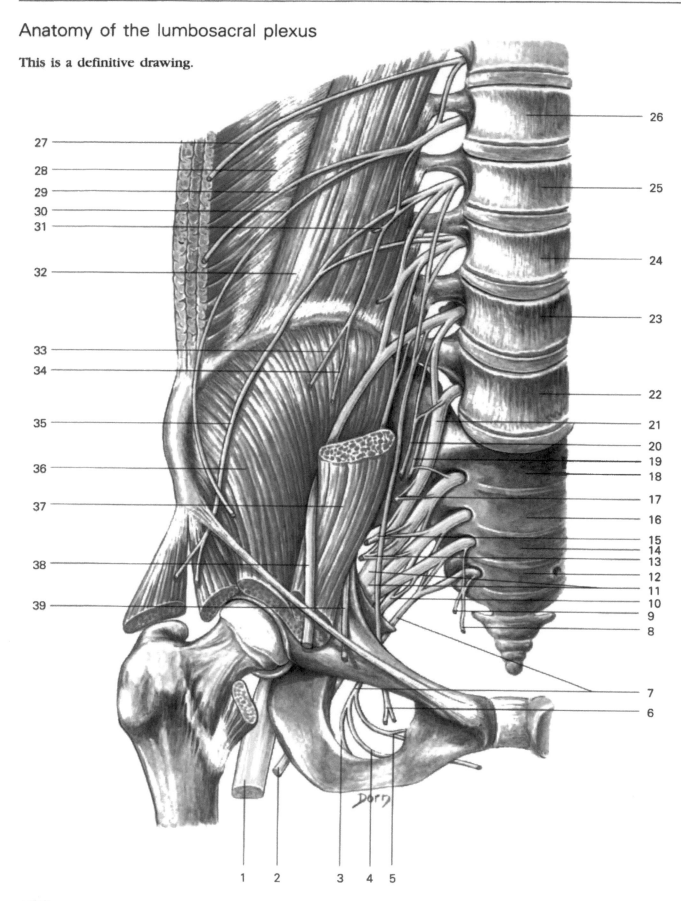

1 sciatic nerve
2 posterior cutaneous nerve of thigh
3 perineal nerve
4 dorsal nerve of penis/clitoris
5 inferior rectal nerve
6 obturator nerve
7 pudendal nerves (S2, 3, 4)
8 perineal branch of fourth sacral nerve
9 to levator ani and coccygeus (S3, 4)
10 posterior cutaneous nerve of thigh (S1, 2, 3)
11 sciatic nerve
12 S4
13 inferior gluteal nerve (L5, S1, 2)
14 S3
15 to piriformis (S1, 2)
16 S2
17 superior gluteal nerve (L4, 5, S1)
18 S1
19 to obturator internus and superior gemellus (L5, S1, 2)
20 to quadratus femoris and inferior gemellus (L5, S1, 2)
21 lumbosacral trunk
22 L5
23 L4
24 L3
25 L2
26 L1
27 subcostal nerve
28 transversus abdominis
29 iliohypogastric nerve (T12, L1)
30 ilioinguinal nerve (L1)
31 to psoas
32 quadratus lumborum
33 femoral branch of genitofemoral nerve
34 genital branch of genitofemoral nerve
35 lateral cutaneous nerve of thigh
36 iliacus
37 psoas
38 femoral nerve (L2, 3, 4)
39 accessory obturator nerve (L3, 4)

Surgery of the knee

Prosthesis of the patella

A Medial approach to the femoropatellar joint.

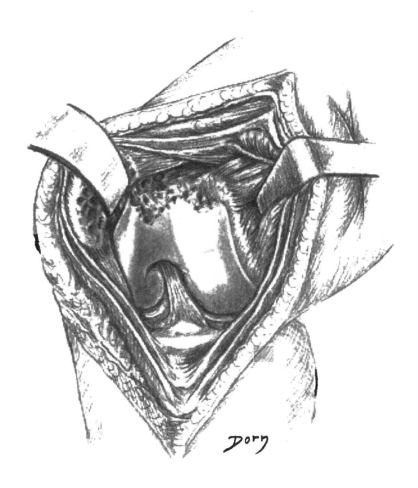

B–D Preparation of the trochlear implant.

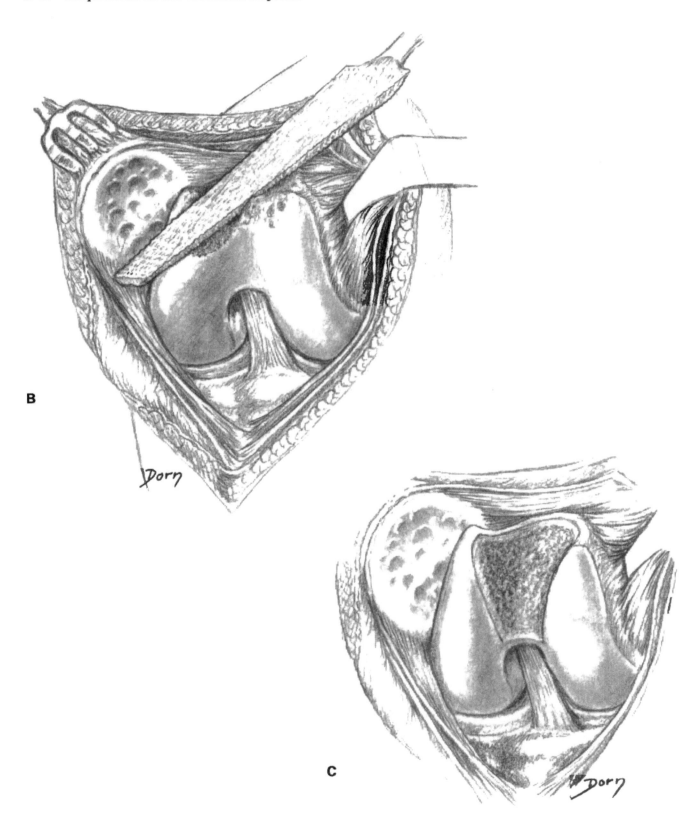

B

C

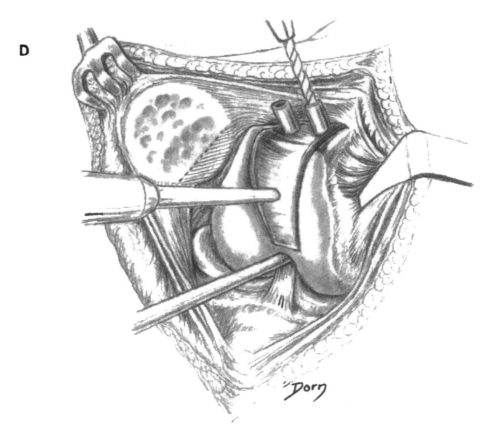

E, F Preparation of the patella.

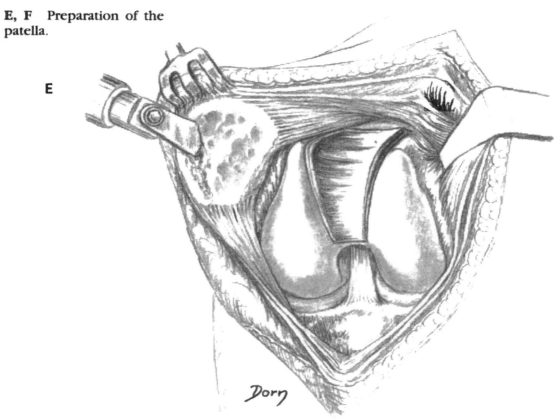

F

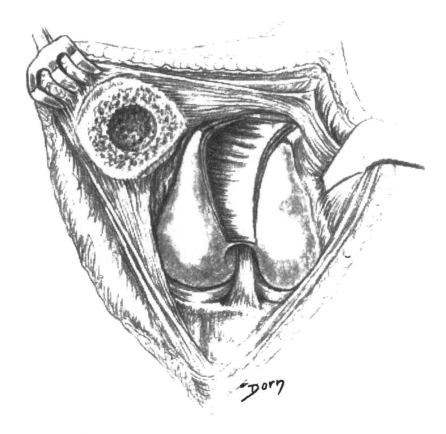

G   The two components are in place.

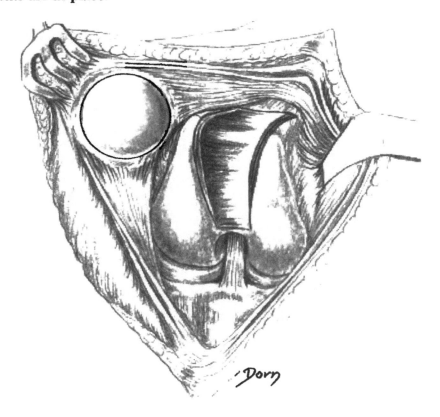

Repair of a rupture of the anterior cruciate ligament

A Anteromedial approach to retrieve the ligament.

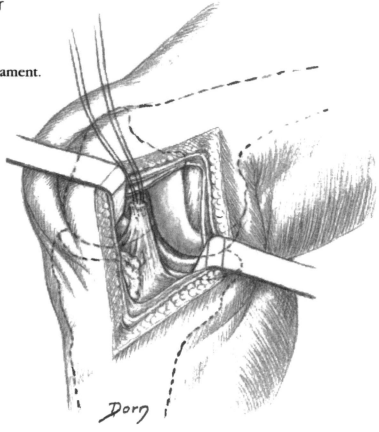

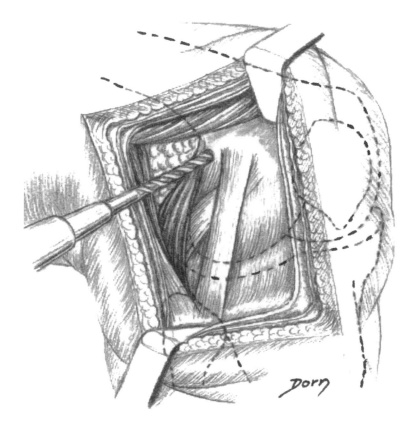

B Posterolateral approach to perform a tunnel 'over the top' of the lateral condyle.

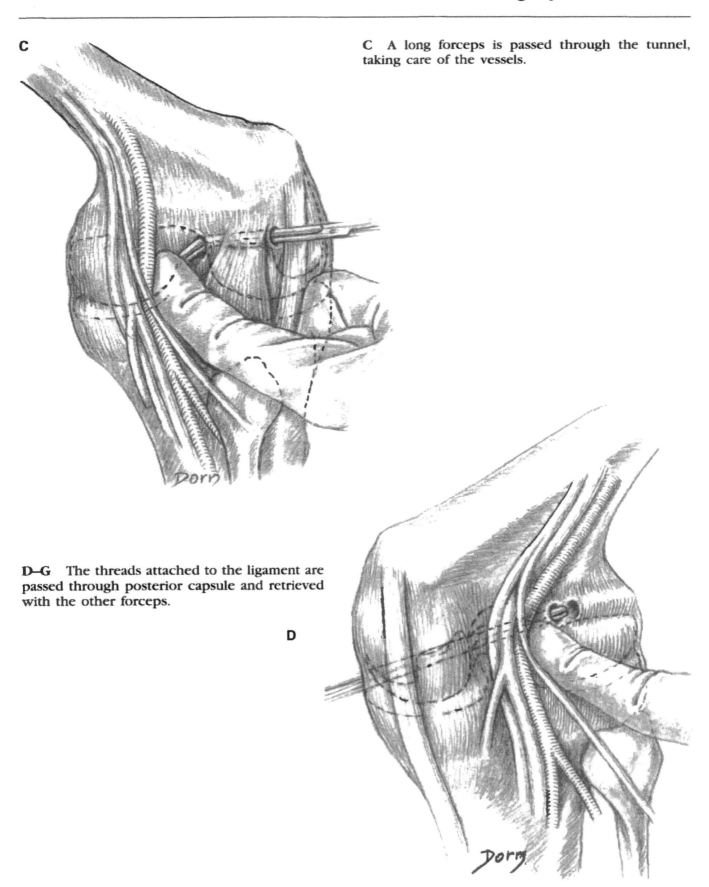

C

C A long forceps is passed through the tunnel, taking care of the vessels.

D–G The threads attached to the ligament are passed through posterior capsule and retrieved with the other forceps.

D

169

E

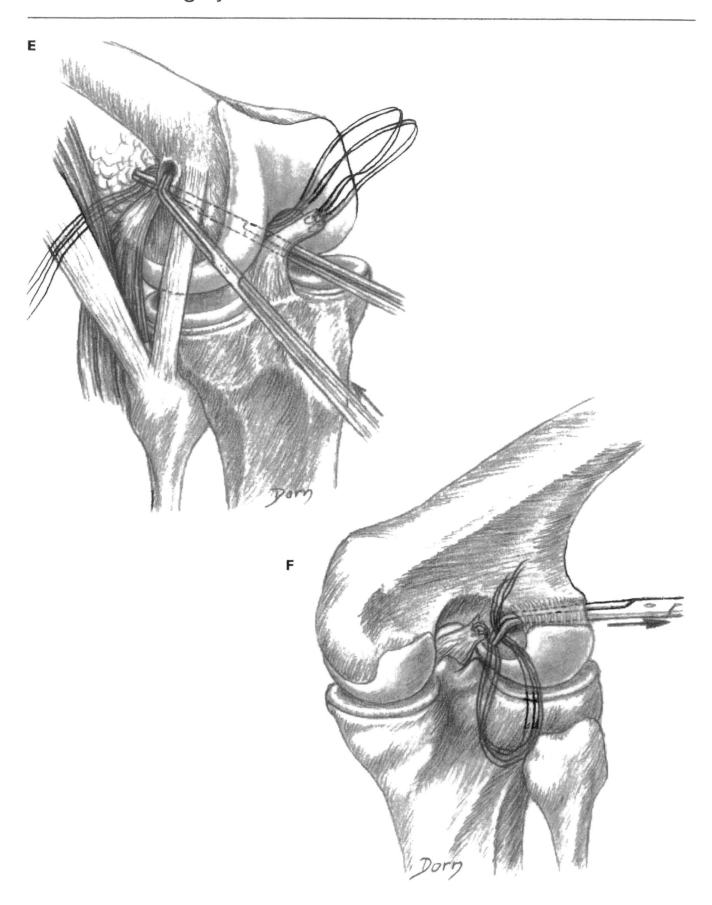

F

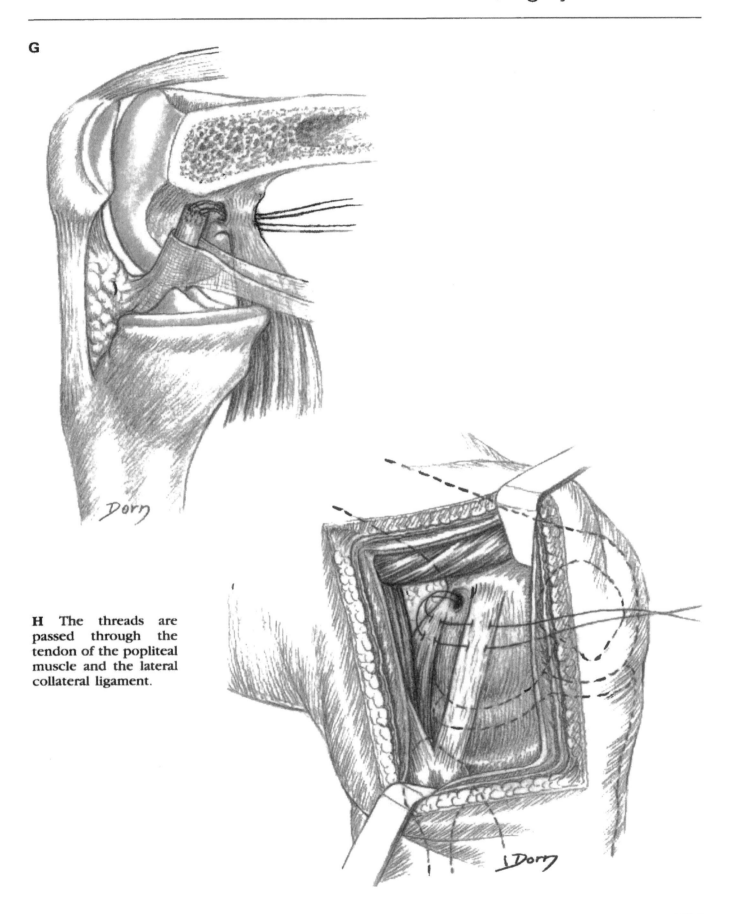

G

H The threads are passed through the tendon of the popliteal muscle and the lateral collateral ligament.

Lower limb surgery

Posterior approach to the posterior cruciate ligament (left limb)

A Popliteal fossa with the medial head of gastrocnemius.

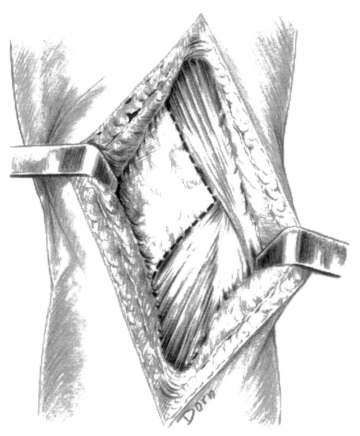

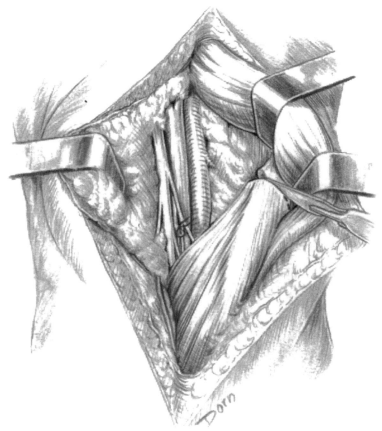

B The tendon of the medial head is divided.

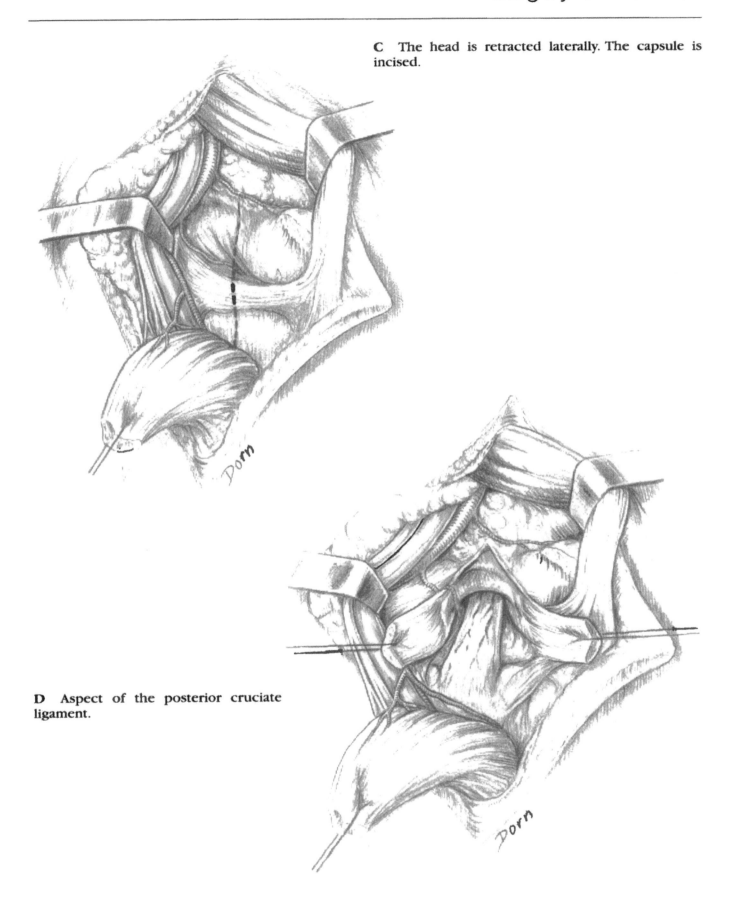

C The head is retracted laterally. The capsule is incised.

D Aspect of the posterior cruciate ligament.

Lower limb surgery

Allograft of patella and patellar ligament

A The continuity of the extensor apparatus is interrupted.

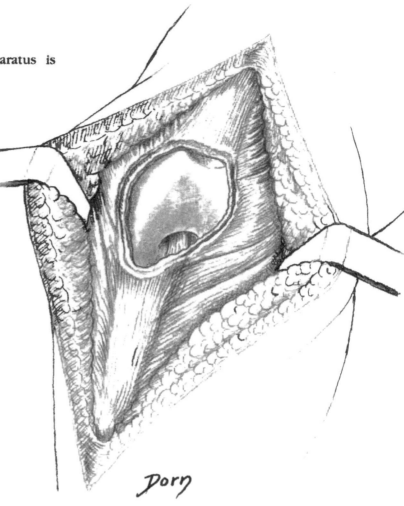

B Preparation of the recipient site.

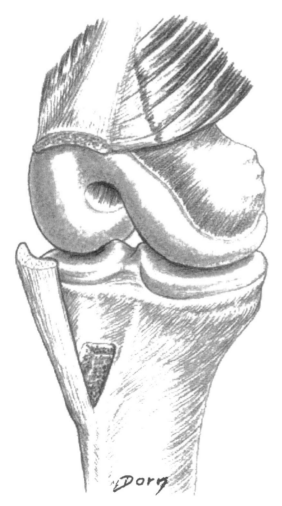

C The allograft with a bone block and a short
portion of rectus femoris tendon.

D Fixation and suture of the allograft.

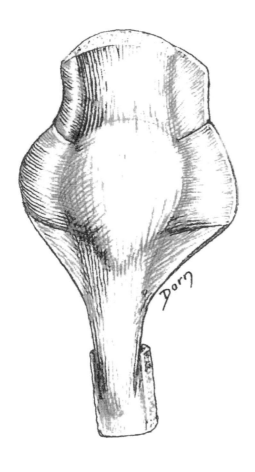

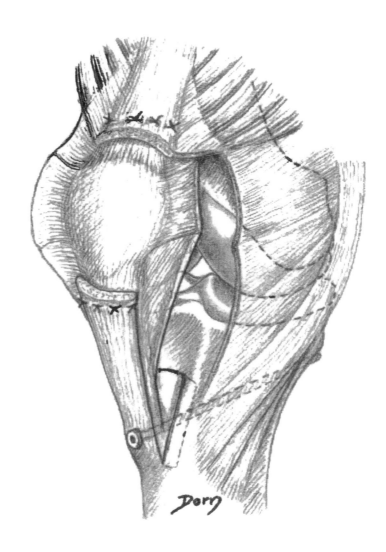

E Final aspect with the sutures of the lateral patellar retinaculi.

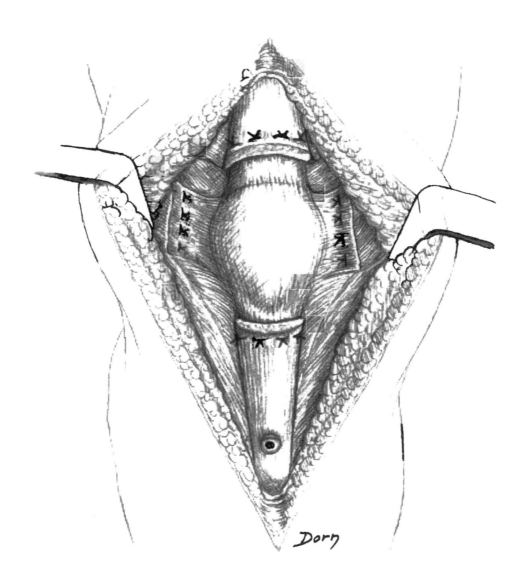

Exposures of the acetabulum

Surgery of the acetabulum is difficult given the depth of the joint and the extensive bone lesions.

Reconstructive surgery of the acetabulum was popularised by R. Judet and E. Letournel. The following series of drawings is among the most beautiful and precise artwork of Léon Dorn.

Cross-section through the hip joint

Note the thick (and unknown) fascia lying at the deep aspect of the rectus femoris.

1 trochanteric bursa
2 obdurator extremis
3 gluteus medius
4 ileopsoas
5 tensor fasciae latae
6 rectus femoris
7 sartorius
8 femoral vessels
9 femoral nerve
10 ilio psoas bursa
11 obturator internus
12 gemellus inferior
13 sciatic nerve

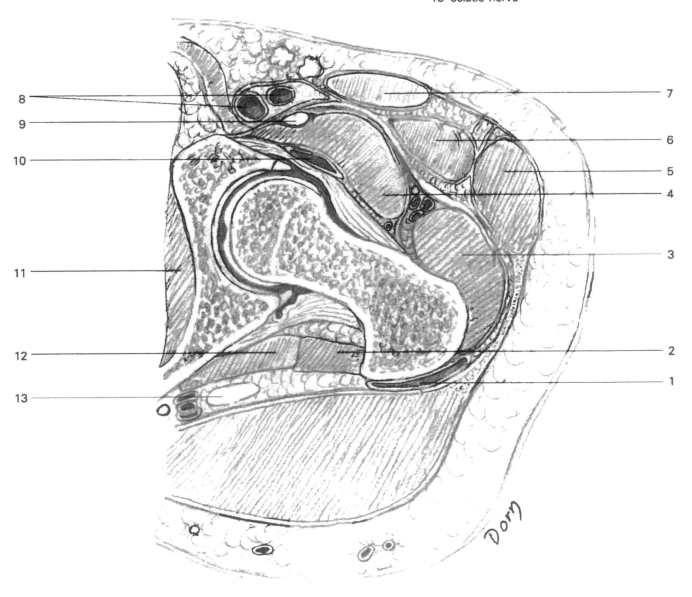

Posterior approach to the acetabulum (Kocher–Langenbeck)

Its indication is the fracture of the posterior wall.

A Skin incision.

B Incision of the iliotibial tract and splitting of the fibres of the gluteus maximum muscle.

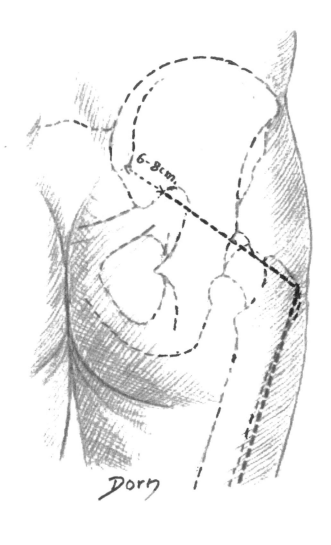

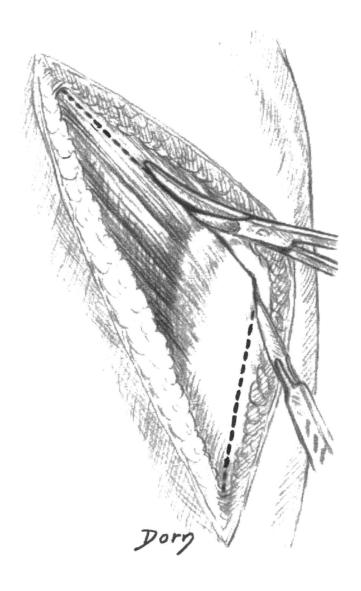

C Exposure of the sciatic nerve and the external rotators of the hip.

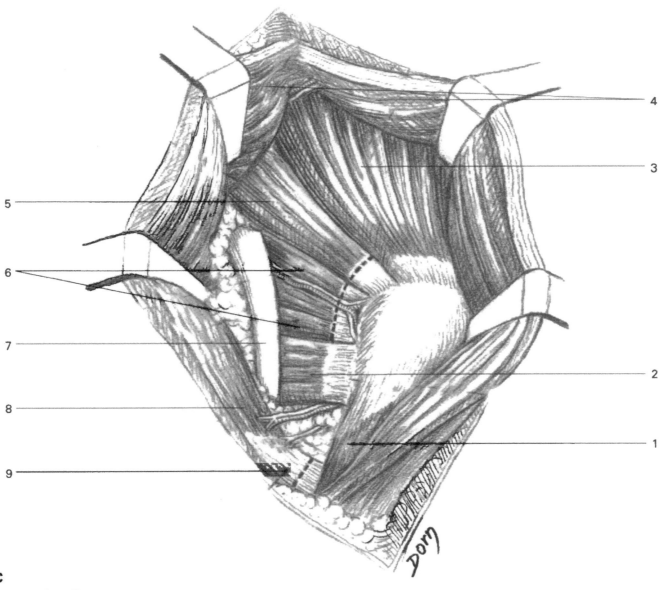

C

1 vastus lateralis
2 quadratus femoris
3 gluteus medius
4 gluteus maximus, split
5 piriformis
6 obturator internis and gemelli
7 sciatic nerve
8 gluteus maximus
9 distal tendon of gluteus maximus (to be cut)

D The rotators are retracted, exposing the capsule; one of the key steps is to find the bursa between the ischium and the obturator internis and the gemelli.

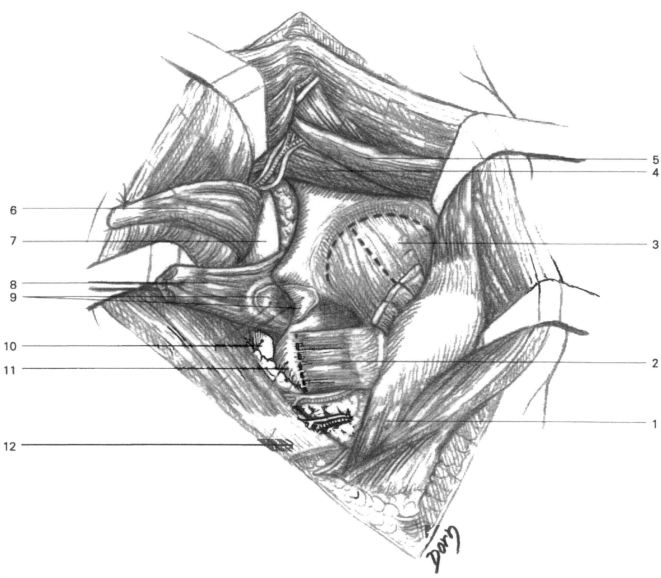

D

1 vastus lateralis
2 quadratus femoris
3 capsule
4 gluteus minimus
5 gluteus medius
6 piriformis
7 sciatic nerve
8 obturator internus and gemelli
9 lesser sciatic notch and bursa
10 sciatic nerve
11 ischion
12 distal tendon of gluteus maximus

E The capsule is incised. Note the retractor which
has been placed into the plane of the bursa.

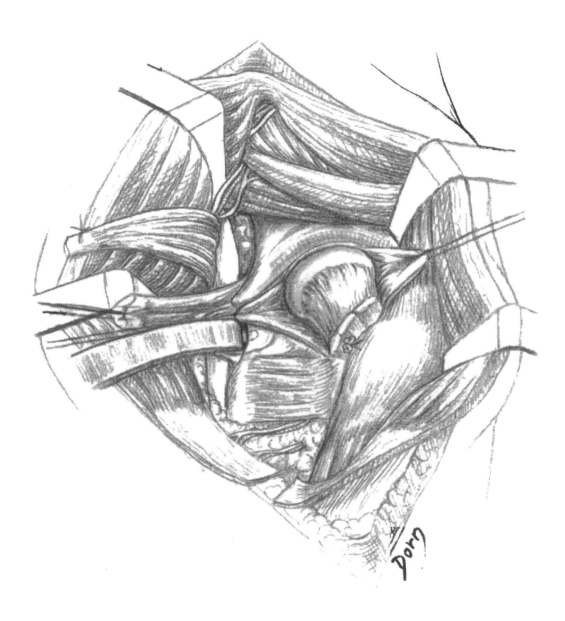

Lower limb surgery

Inguinal approach to the acetabulum

Its indications are the fracture of anterior wall or anterior column and some complex fractures involving both columns of the acetabulum.

A The fascia is incised in line with the skin incision.

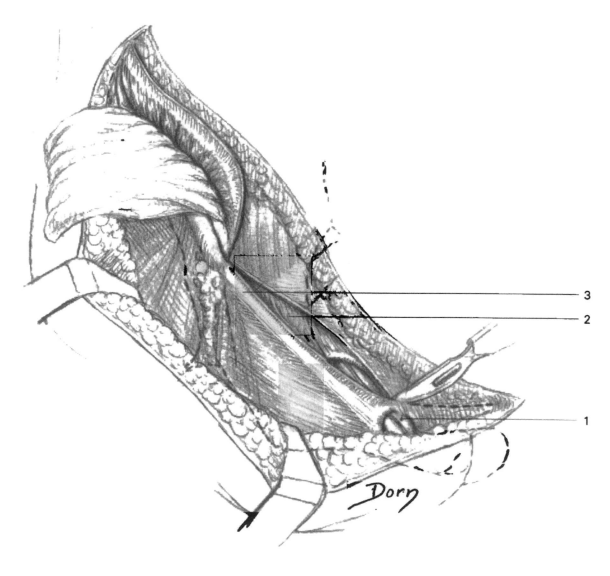

A

1 spermatic cord
2 internal oblique
3 inguinal ligament

182

B The spermatic cord, the external iliac vessels, the femoral nerve, the psoas muscle and the lateral cutaneous nerve of the thigh have been isolated. The iliopsoas fascia is severed.

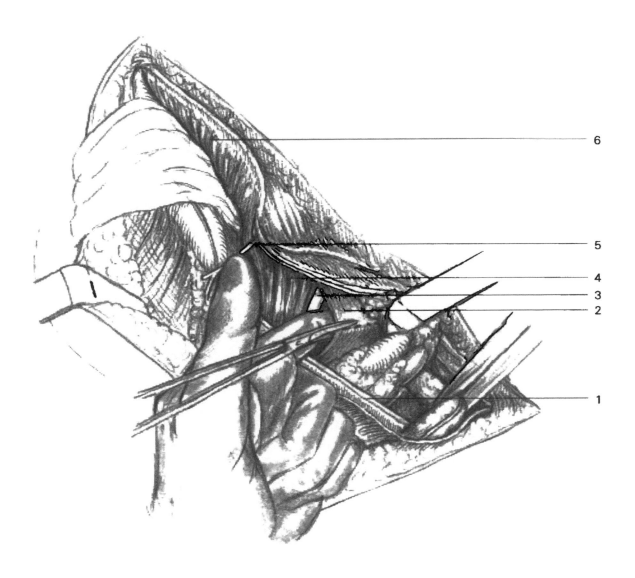

B

1 inguinal ligament
2 iliopsoas fascia
3 femoral nerve
4 iliopsoas
5 lateral cutaneous nerve of thigh
6 iliacus

Lower limb surgery

C All the structures are held and retracted by rubber slings. Medial retraction of the iliopsoas provides access to the iliac fossa.

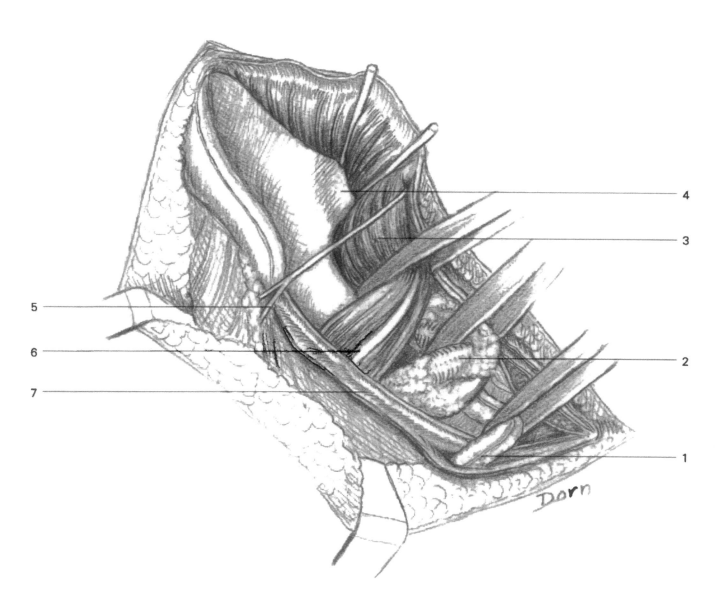

C

1 spermatic cord
2 external iliac vessels sheath
3 ilio psoas
4 sacroiliac joint
5 lateral cutaneous nerve of the thigh
6 femoral nerve
7 inguinal ligament

D Lateral retraction of the iliopsoas gives access to the pelvic brim.

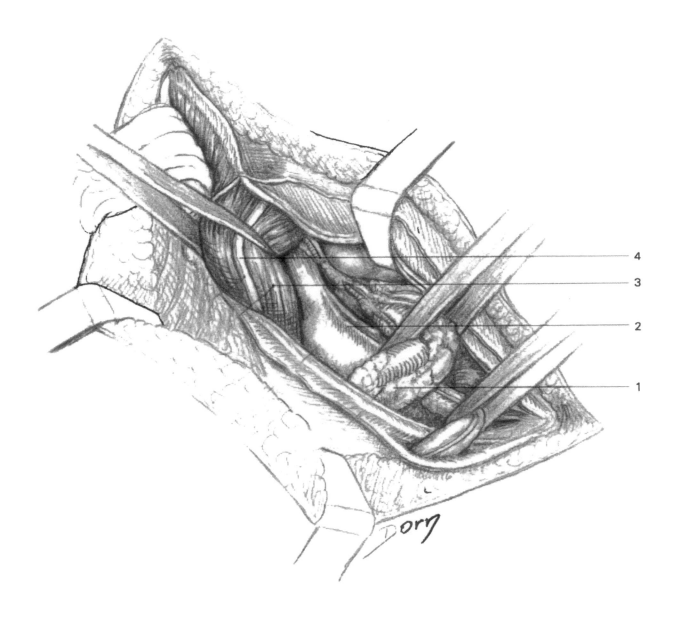

4
3
2
1

D

1 external iliac vessels
2 ilio pectineal eminence
3 ilio psoas
4 femoral nerve

E Lateral retraction of the vessels and spermatic cord gives access to the superior pubic ramus.

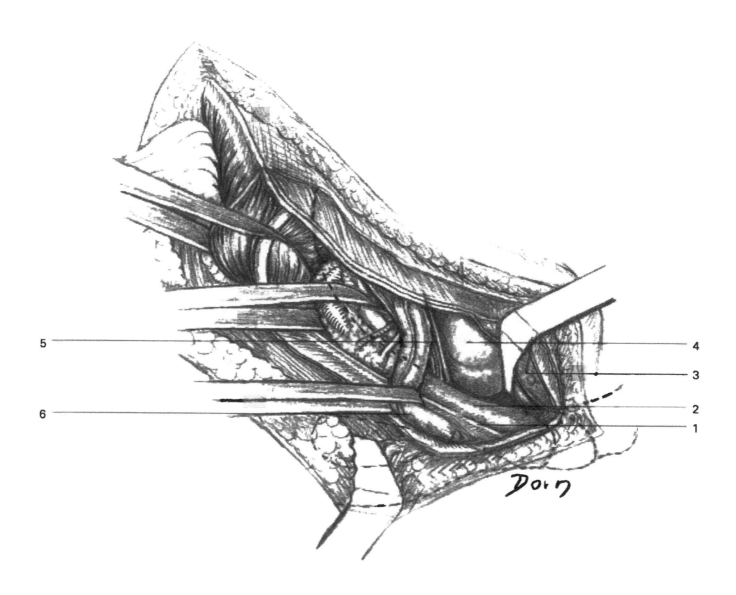

5   4

        3

6   2

        1

E

1 inguinal ligament
2 superior pubic rami
3 rectus abdominus
4 urinary bladder
5 neurovascular obturator bundle
6 spermatic cord

Extended iliofemoral approach to the acetabulum

This approach is also indicated in fractures of both columns.

A The gluteal muscles are reflected from the external iliac wing.

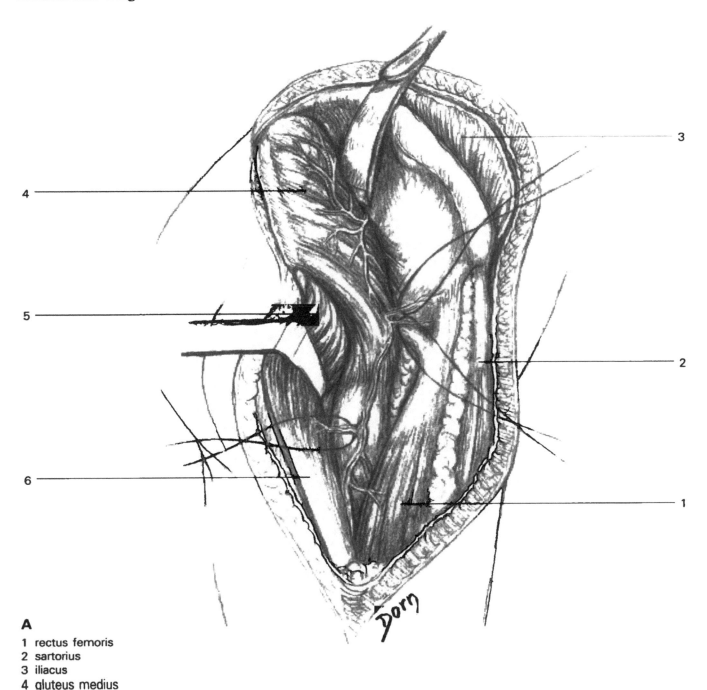

A
1 rectus femoris
2 sartorius
3 iliacus
4 gluteus medius
5 tensor fasciae latae
6 fascia lata

B The insertions of gluteus minimus and gluteus medius have been divided. The massive muscular flap comprising the gluteal muscles and tensor fascia latae is retracted posteriorly, exposing the short external rotators.

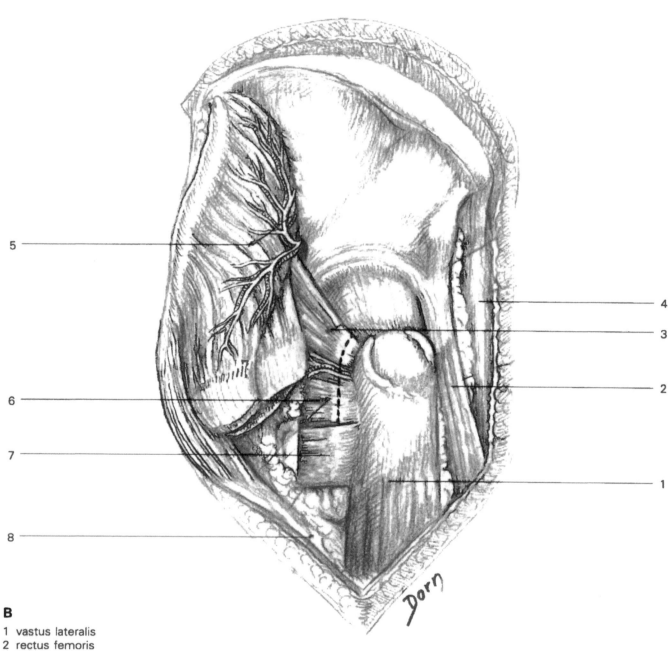

B

1 vastus lateralis
2 rectus femoris
3 piriformis
4 sartorius
5 gluteus medius
6 pelvitrochanteric muscles
7 quadratus femoris
8 distal tendon of gluteus maximus

C The short rotators have been divided and retracted. Retraction of the piriformis exposes the sciatic nerve. The whole acetabulum is visible.

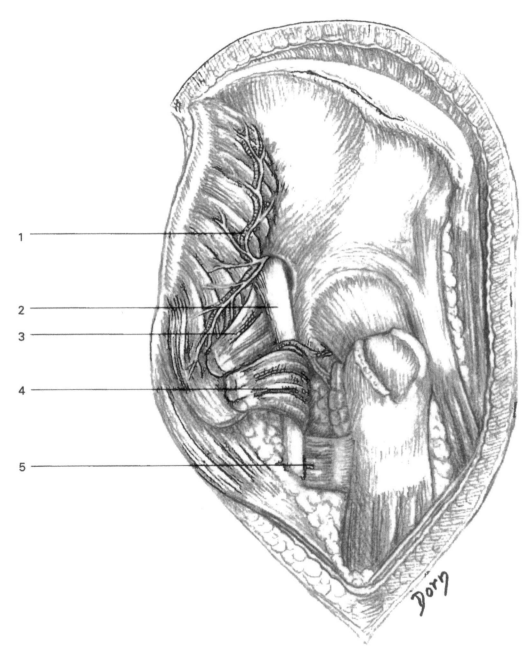

C

1 superior gluteal pedicle and nerve
2 sciatic nerve
3 piriformis
4 obturator internus and the gemelli
5 quadratus femoris

D Elevation of the iliacus, sartorius and inguinal ligament gives access to the internal iliac fossa.

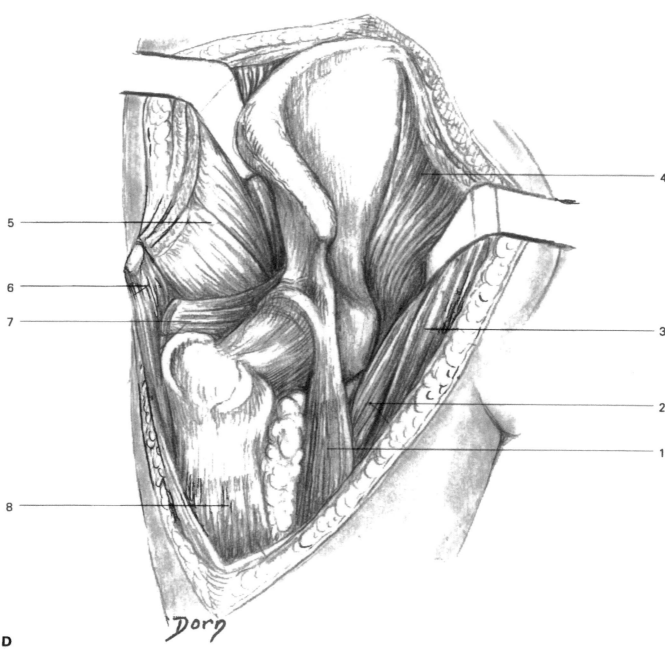

D

1 rectus femoris
2 iliopsoas
3 sartorius
4 iliacus
5 glutei
6 tensor fasciae latae
7 piriformis
8 vastus lateralis

Approaches to the foot and ankle

Posteromedial approach to the ankle

A, B Skin incision. The flexor retinaculum is incised in line with the skin. The neurovascular bundle is identified.

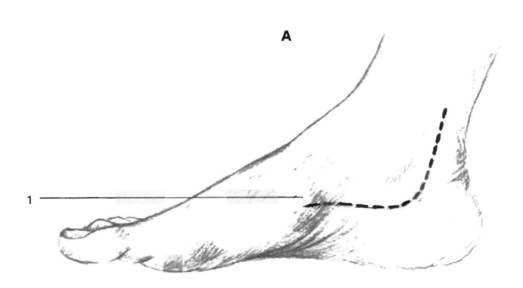

A

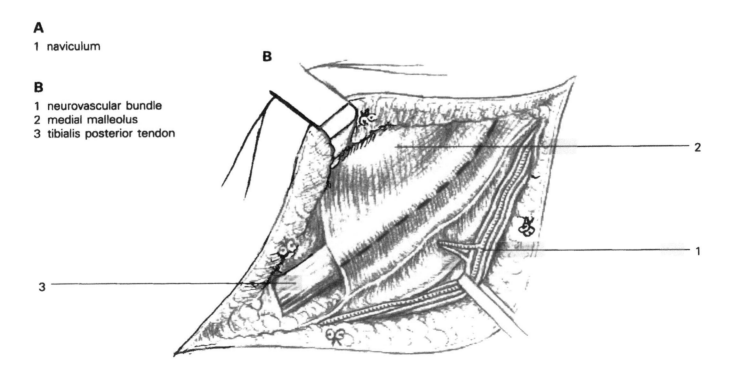

A
1 naviculum

B
1 neurovascular bundle
2 medial malleolus
3 tibialis posterior tendon

C The tendon of tibialis posterior is retracted anteriorly exposing the deltoid ligament.

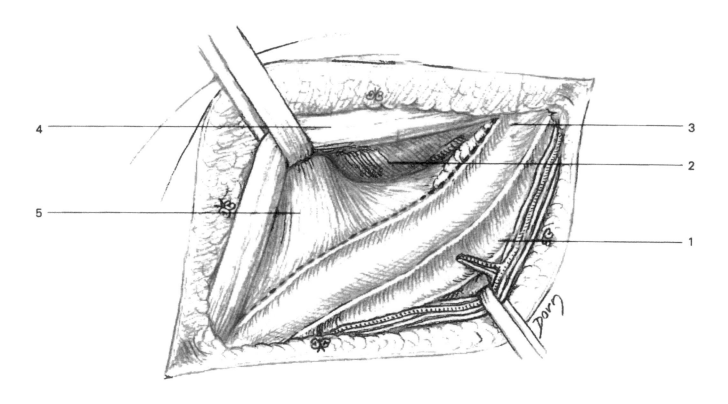

C

1 neurovascular bundle sheath
2 malleolus medialis
3 tendon of flexor digitorum longus within its sheath
4 tibialis posterior tendon
5 deltoid ligament

D The capsule is incised, giving access to the subtalar joint and the posterior aspect of the ankle, chiefly if Achilles' tendon has been divided.

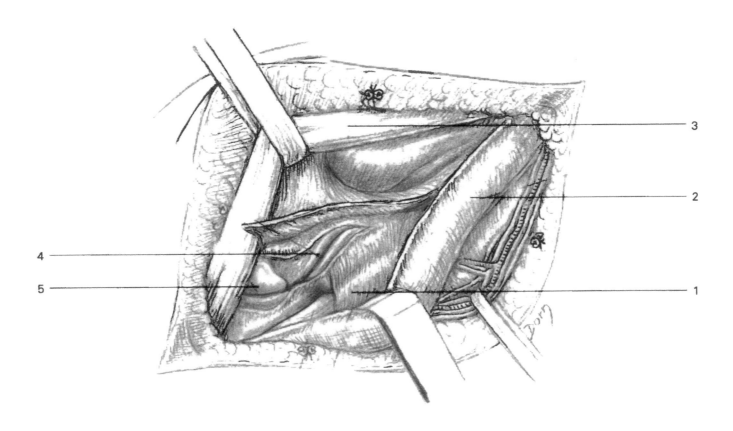

D

1 flexor hallucis longus
2 flexor digitorum longus retracted
3 tibialis posterior tendon
4 subtalar joint
5 head of talus

Lateral approach to the subtalar and midtarsal joint

This exposure is used for fusion of the joints.

A, B Skin incision, exposing the inferior extensor retinaculum.

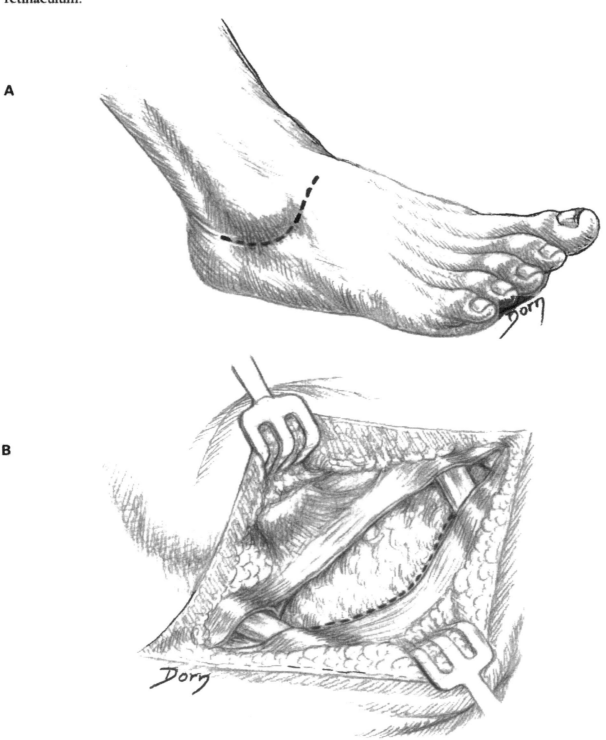

C The extensor digitorum brevis muscle is detached to expose the subtalar joint.

C

1 calcaneum
2 extensor digitorum brevis
3 anterior tibiofibular ligament
4 fibula
5 calcaneo fibular ligament
6 talus

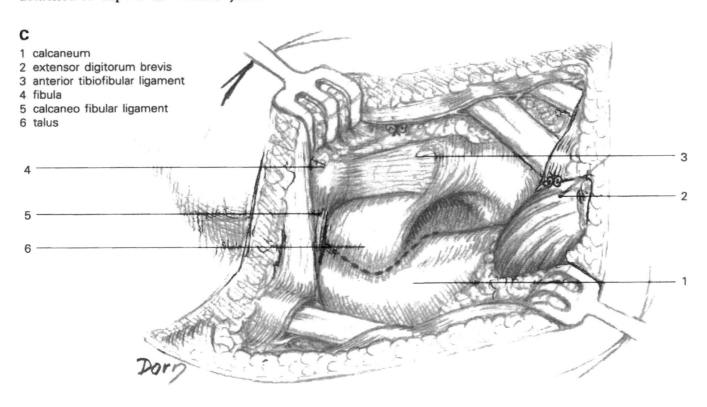

D The subtalar joint and the talonavicular and calcaneocuboid joints are exposed.

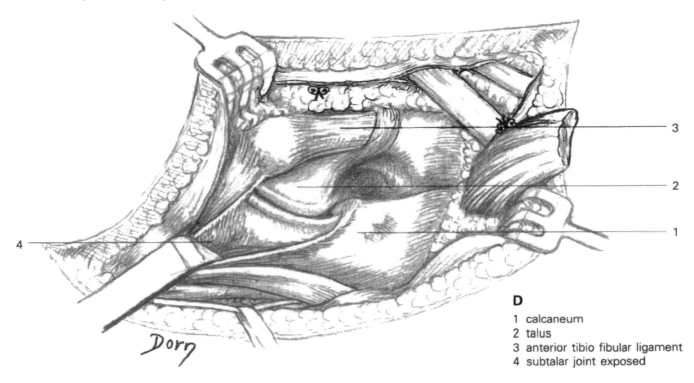

D

1 calcaneum
2 talus
3 anterior tibio fibular ligament
4 subtalar joint exposed

9

Miscellaneous

Muscular studies

The shape of the human body is very attractive for a medical illustrator.

Studies of the muscular relief were one of the main interests of the artists of the Renaissance. It can be said that one of the motivations for dissection during this period was to understand how the muscles contribute to the shape of the body. The following drawings of Léon Dorn, particularly the first one, recall the 'écorché of Vésale'. The difference is that Vésale's man seems to be very anxious while Dorn's has a relaxed (modern) attitude.

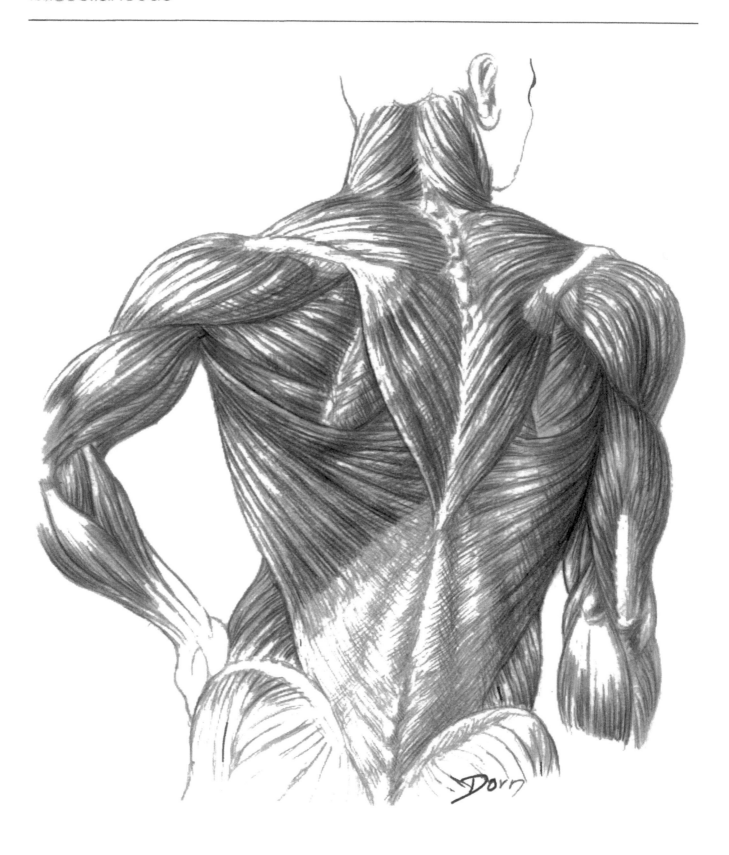

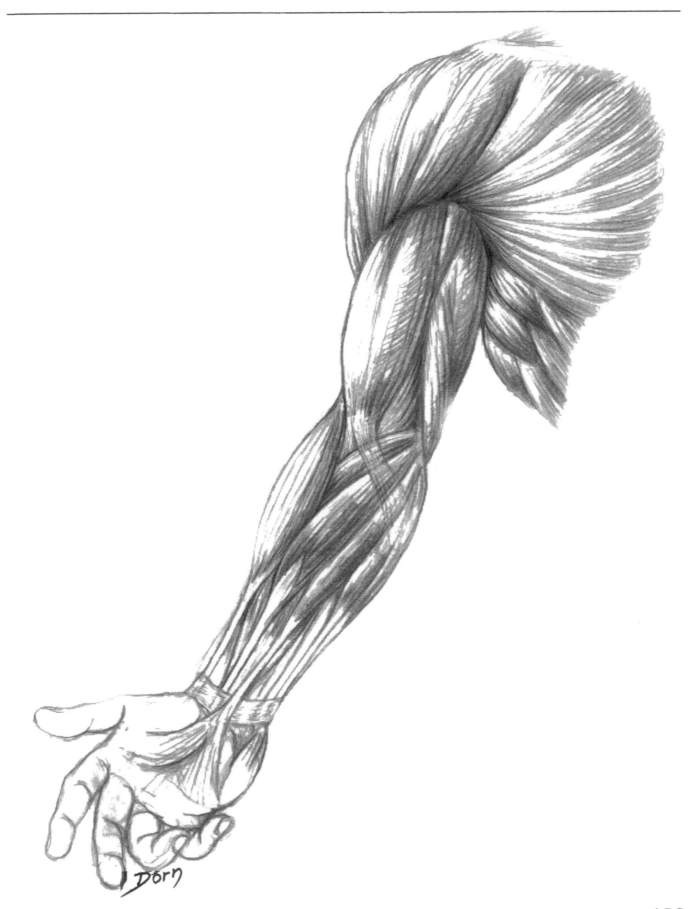

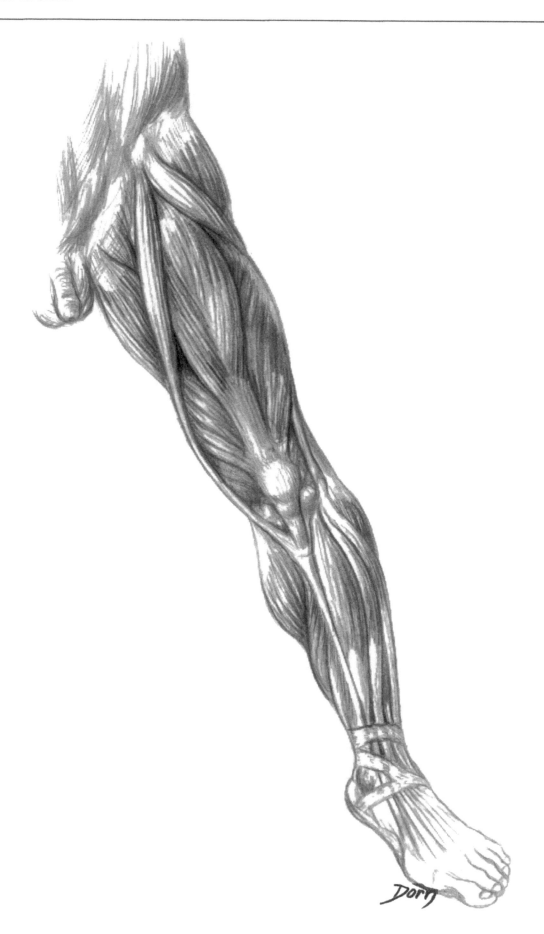

Surgery of the ear

A series of drawings showing the boundary between neurosurgery and ear surgery

The first three drawings are devoted to the approach through the skull. The dura mater has been opened which allows exposure of the facial and other nerves.

A Exposure of a tumour of the vestibular nerve by a retroauricular and transvestibular approach.

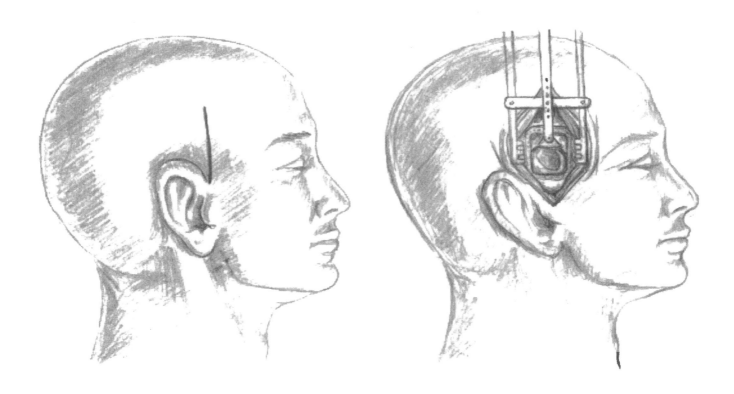

B Opening of the endolymphatic sac in a case of
Ménière's disease.

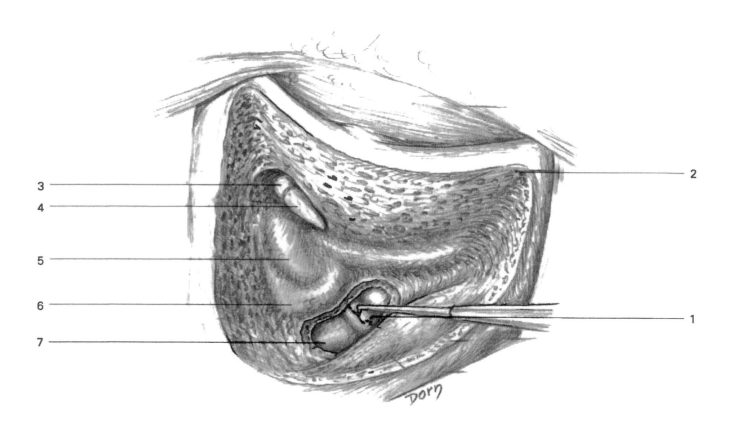

B

1 opening of the endolymphatic sac
2 mastoid cortex
3 malleus (head of malleus)
4 incus (short process)
5 lateral semicircular canal
6 posterior semicircular canal
7 stripped cerebellum dura mater

C Transmastoid approach to expose the second and third parts of the facial nerve, which is taken out of the Fallopian aqueduct.

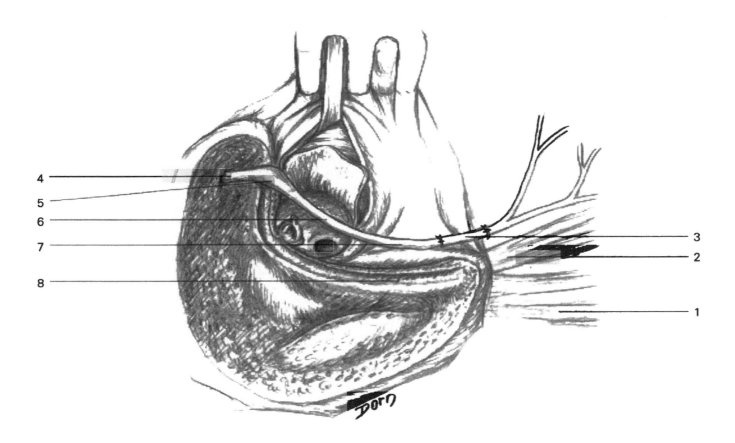

C

1 sternocleidomastoid muscle
2 digastric muscle
3 facial nerve grafting
4 labrynthine segment of the facial nerve
5 gerniculate ganglion of the facial nerve
6 tympanic segment of the facial nerve
7 mastoid segment of the facial nerve
8 empty Fallopian aqueduct

Surgery of the middle ear

A The transmeatal and extended transmeatal approaches to the middle ear, which allows harvesting a temporal fascia graft.

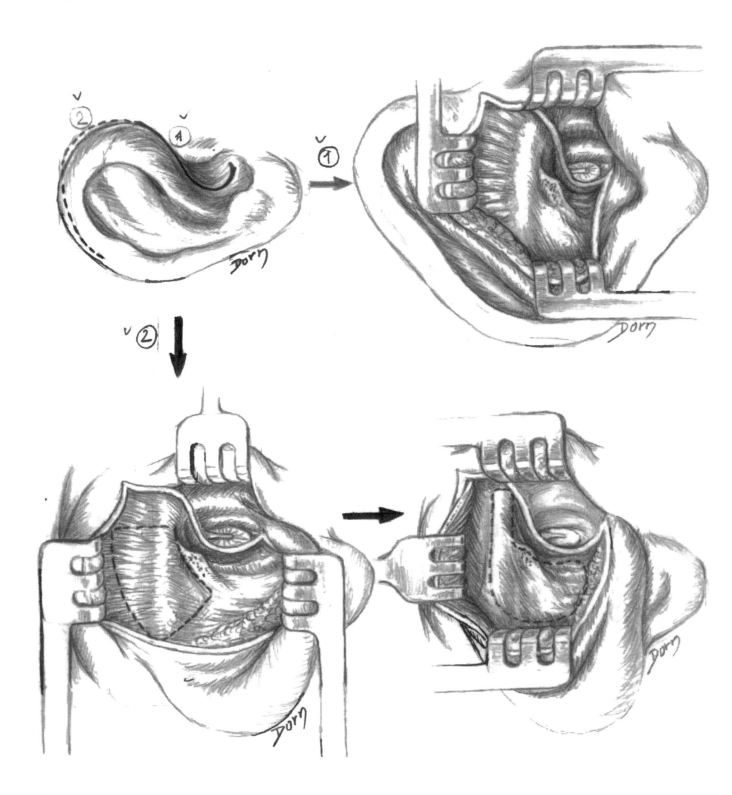

B The Shambaugh approach allows grooving of the cavities of the middle ear.

B

1 relief of sigmoid sinus
2 antium opened
3 lateral semicircular canal
4 anterior epitypanum
5 facial nerve
6 canal wall skin

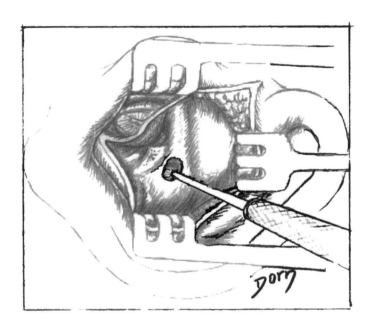

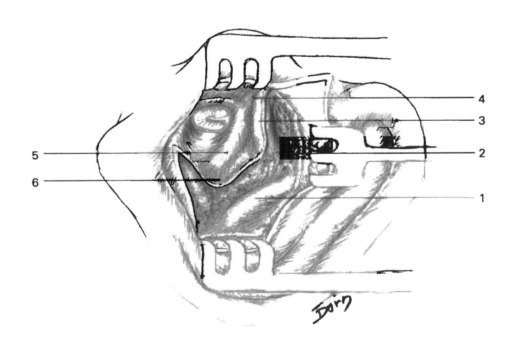

Miscellaneous

Tympanic graft

A Mastoidectomy (canal wall up procedure).

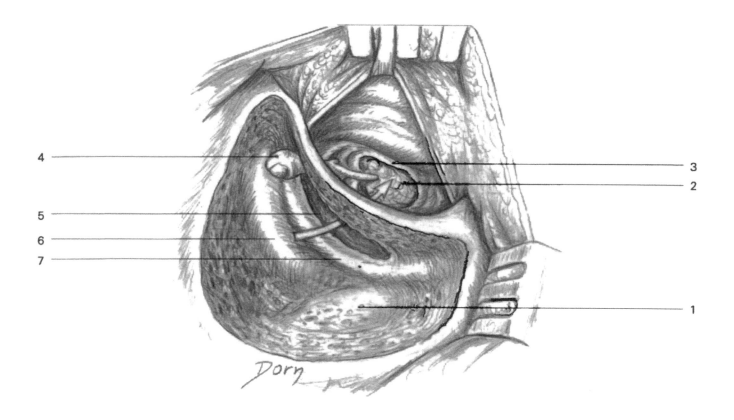

A

1 sigmoid sinus
2 cholesteatoma
3 perforated tympanic membrane
4 head of the malleus
5 posterior tympanectomy (facial recess opened)
6 lateral semicircular canal
7 facial nerve

B Exploration of the tympanic cavity, sparing the facial nerve. Mastoidectomy (canal wall down procedure) with tympanoplasty.

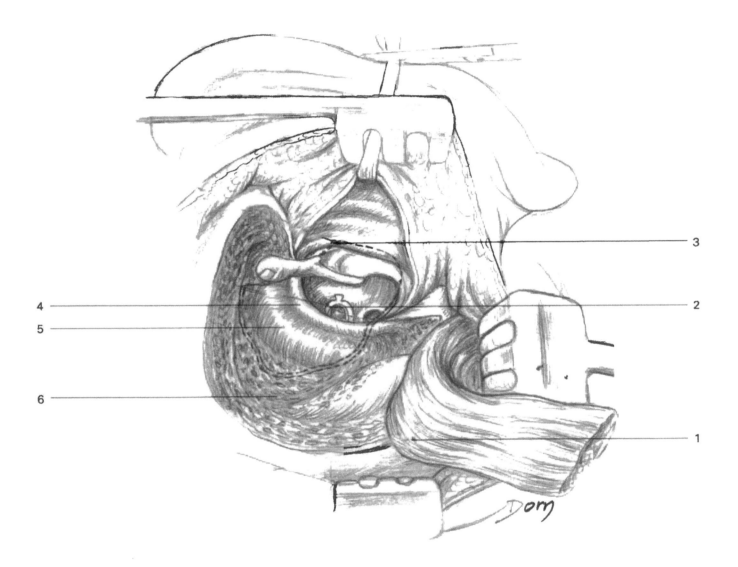

A

1 fibromuscular flap raised from the mastoidian and temporal muscles
2 stapes
3 temporal aponeurosis graft under the tympanic rests, on the facial nerve and the lateral semicircular canal
4 facial nerve
5 lateral semicircular canal
6 automastoidian cavity

C A muscular flap from the temporal muscle fills up the mastoid cavity. Reconstruction of the auditory canal.

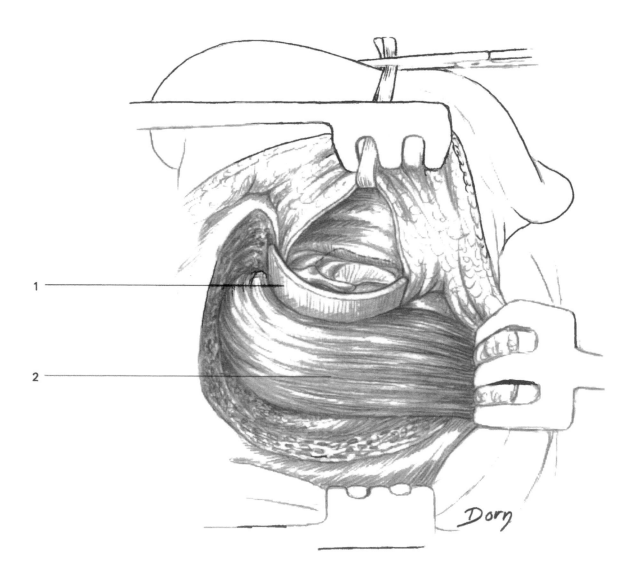

c

1 temporal aponeurosis graft prefigures the final outer ear canal
2 fascia temporalis graft and muscular flap of the temporalis muscle

Paediatrics

Crying baby with a Pavlick's harness
to prevent hip dislocation or instability

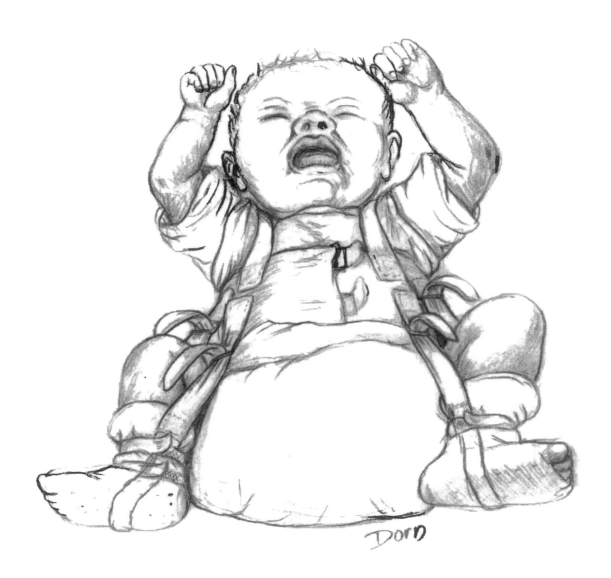

Miscellaneous

Congenital malformations

Each plate shows the relation of the clinical aspect with the anatomical lesions and the ultrasound imaging aspect

A   Myelomeningocele.

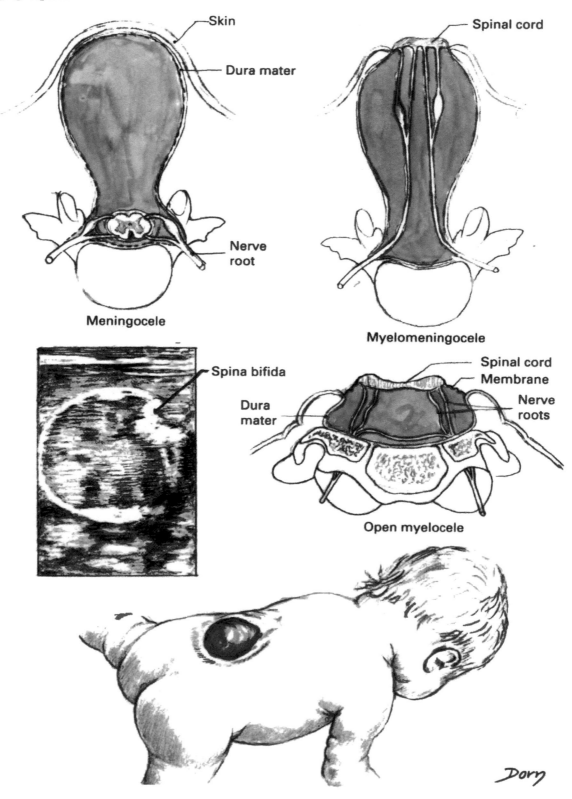

Skin

Dura mater

Nerve root

Meningocele

Spinal cord

Myelomeningocele

Spina bifida

Dura mater

Spinal cord
Membrane

Nerve roots

Open myelocele

Dory

B Laparoschisis.

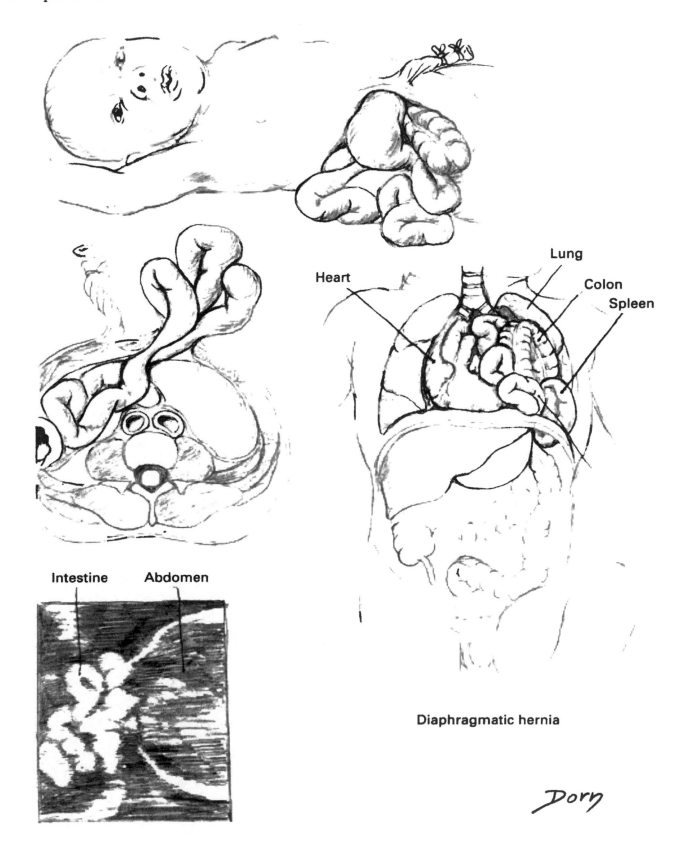

Intestine   Abdomen

Heart   Lung   Colon   Spleen

Diaphragmatic hernia

Dorn

C   Cystic tumour of the lungs.

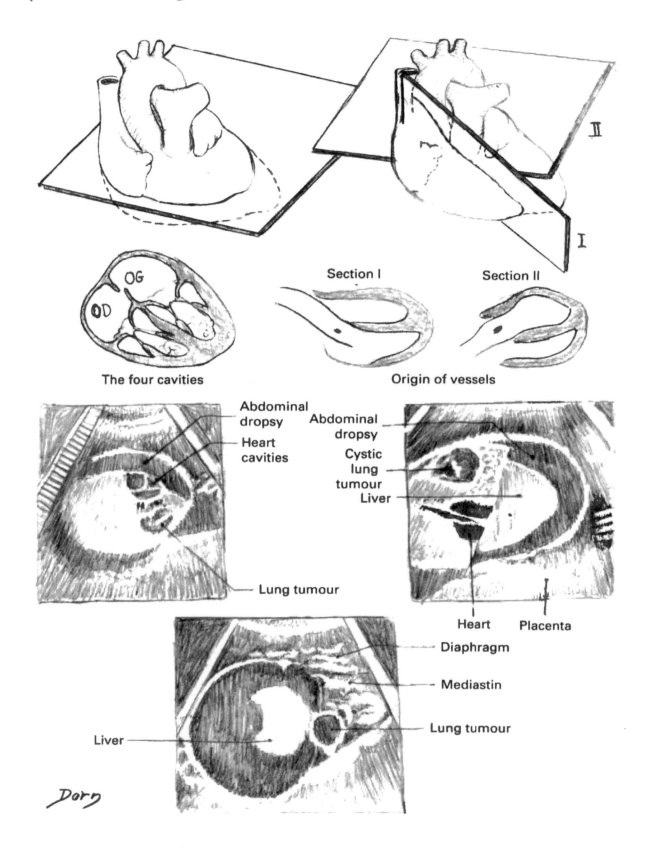

The four cavities

Section I

Section II

Origin of vessels

Abdominal dropsy

Heart cavities

Lung tumour

Abdominal dropsy

Cystic lung tumour

Liver

Heart   Placenta

Diaphragm

Mediastin

Lung tumour

Liver

Dorn

D Different varieties of tumours: cystic hygroma; lymphangioma; sacrococcygeal teratoma.

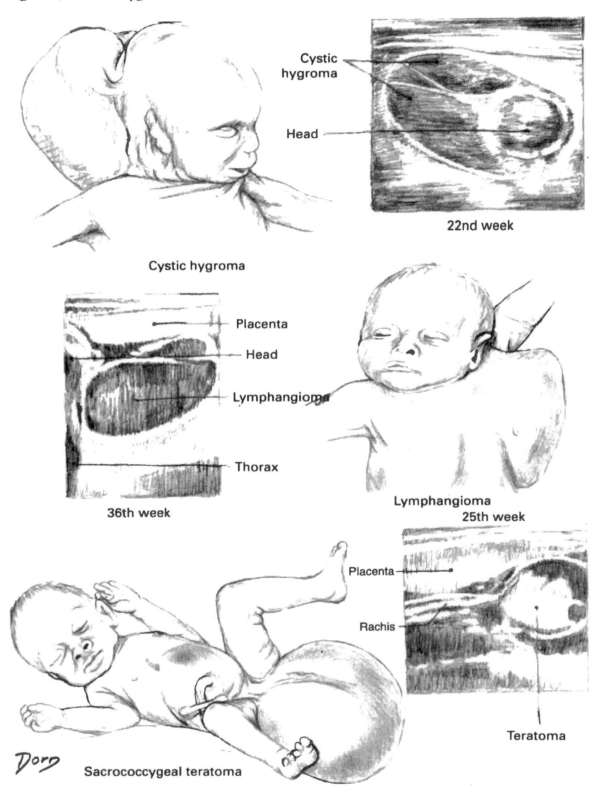

Cystic hygroma

22nd week

Cystic hygroma

36th week

Lymphangioma
25th week

Sacrococcygeal teratoma

E Anomalies of the urinary tract: agenesis of the kidneys; cystic tumour of the kidneys.

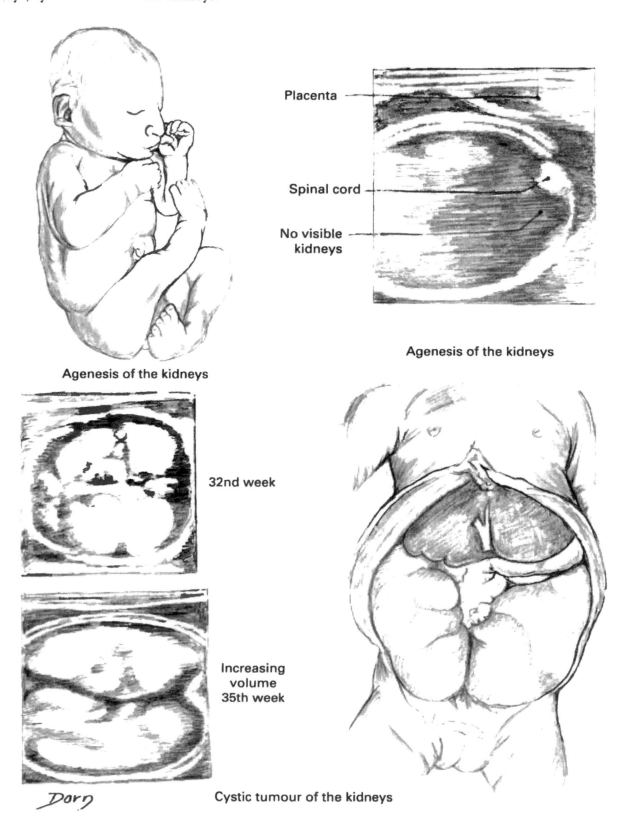

Agenesis of the kidneys

Placenta

Spinal cord

No visible kidneys

Agenesis of the kidneys

32nd week

Increasing volume 35th week

Dorn

Cystic tumour of the kidneys

F Achondrogenesis.

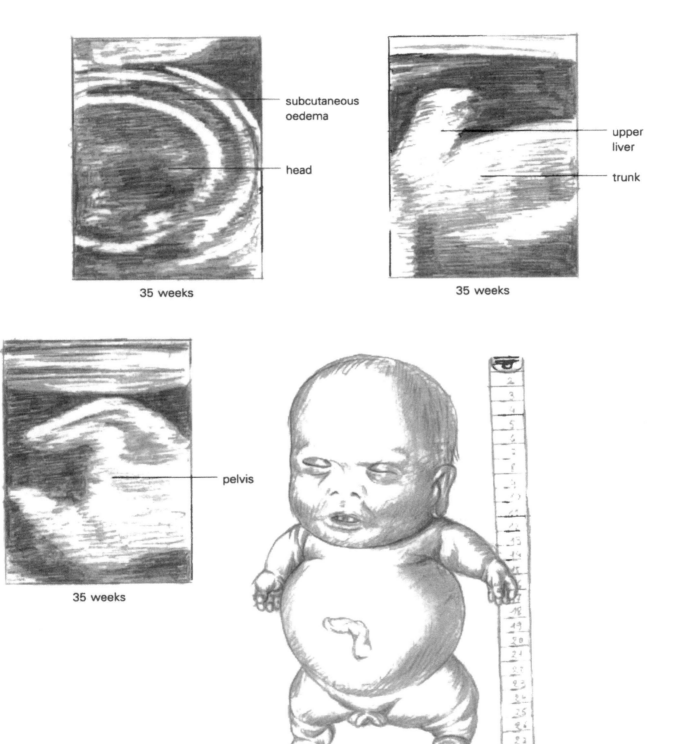

subcutaneous oedema

head

35 weeks

upper liver

trunk

35 weeks

pelvis

35 weeks

Dorn

Achondrogenesis

Miscellaneous

G Omphalocele.

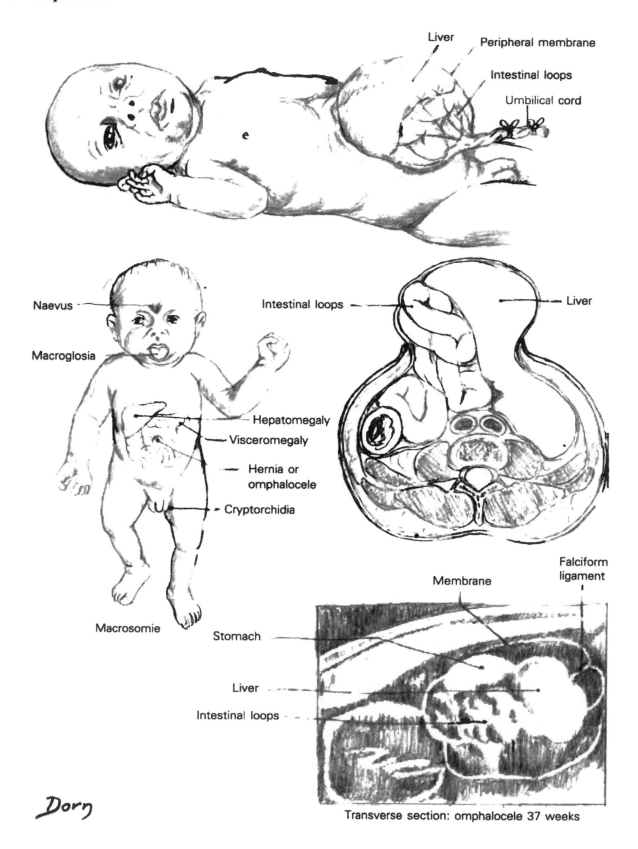

Liver
Peripheral membrane
Intestinal loops
Umbilical cord

Naevus
Macroglosia

Intestinal loops
Liver

Hepatomegaly
Visceromegaly
Hernia or omphalocele
Cryptorchidia

Macrosomie

Stomach
Liver
Intestinal loops

Membrane
Falciform ligament

Dorn

Transverse section: omphalocele 37 weeks

H Monstrous anomalies.

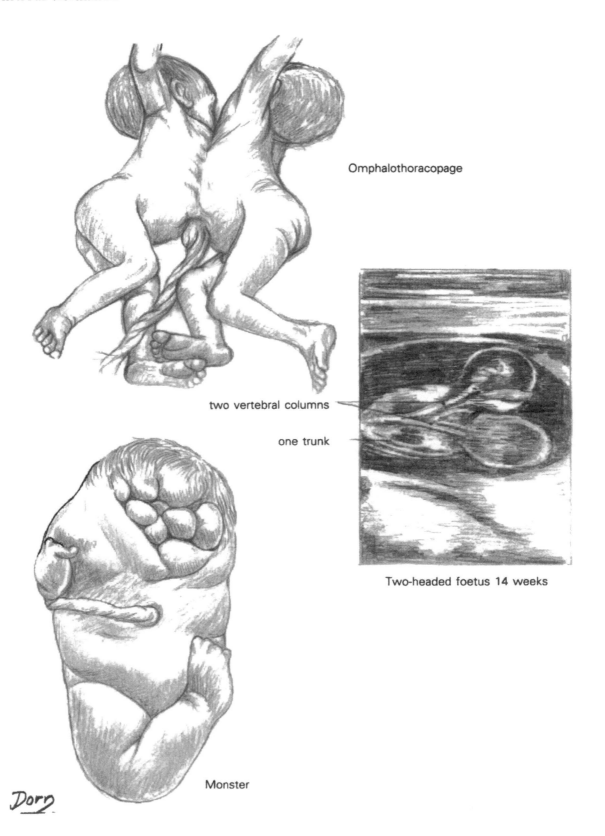

Omphalothoracopage

two vertebral columns

one trunk

Two-headed foetus 14 weeks

Monster

Detection of fetal anomalies.
Amniocentesis under ultrasound
imaging

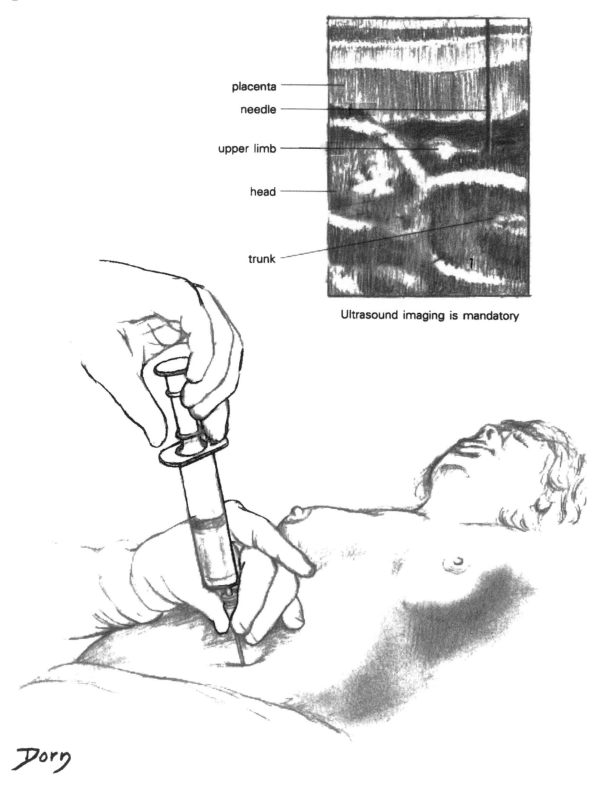

placenta
needle

upper limb

head

trunk

Ultrasound imaging is mandatory

Dorn

Heart anatomy

Heart anatomy cannot be understood without exposing the cavities.

Dissection of the left heart

A Section of the left auricle between the two pulmonary veins.

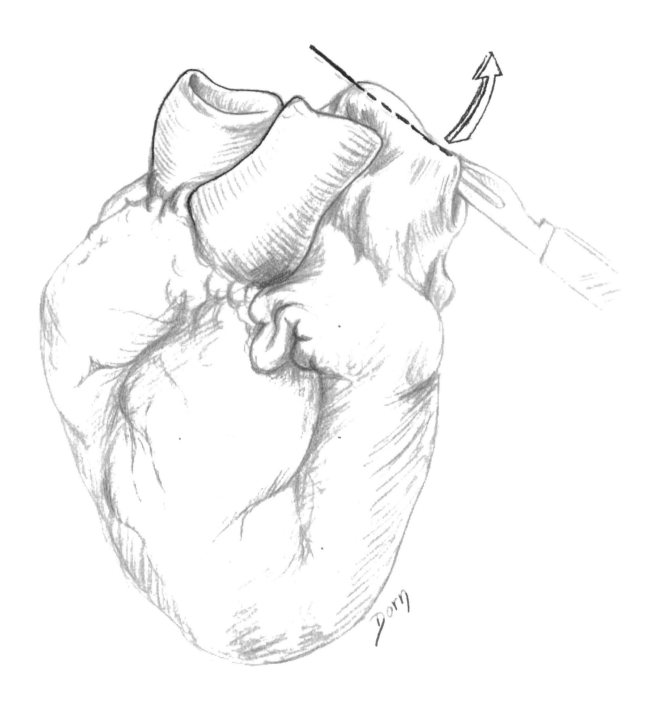

B The knife is introduced in the left auricle.

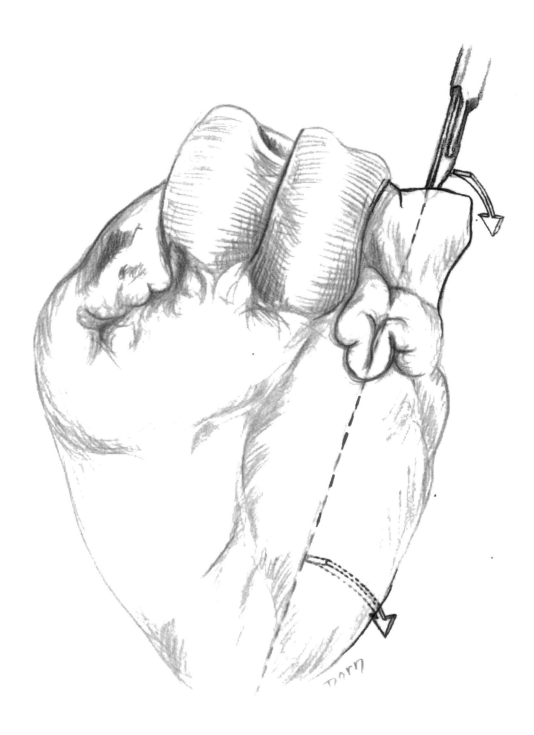

C   Left ventricle. The mitral valve and the anterior
and posterior papillary muscles are visible.

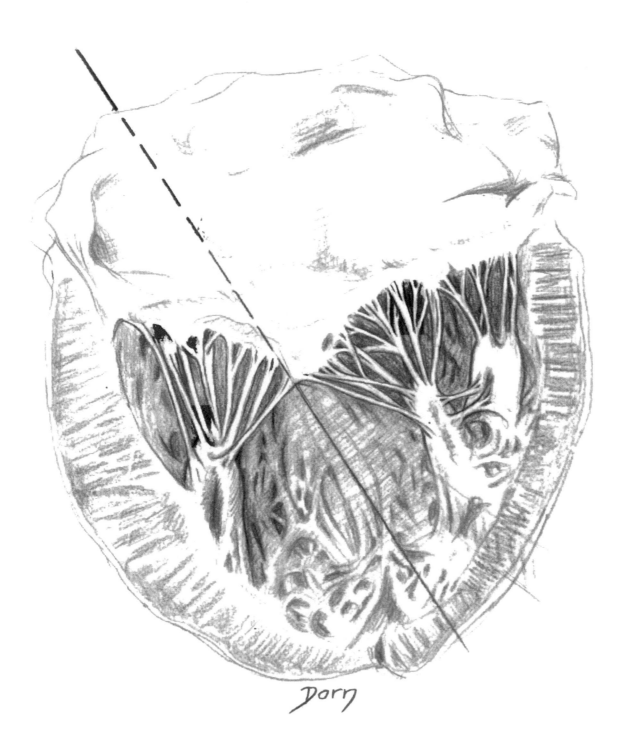

Dorn

D The left ventricle is separated into two parts.

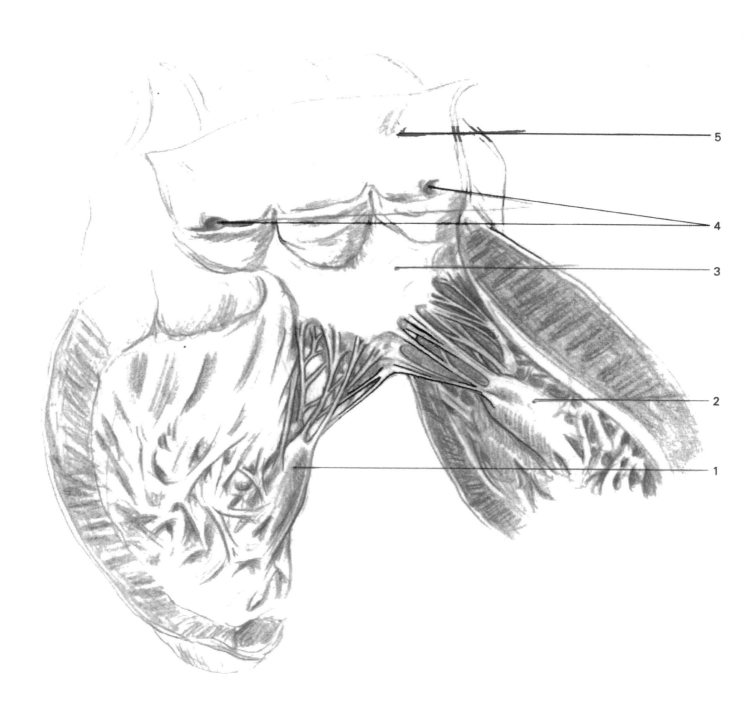

D

1 posterior papillary muscle
2 anterior papillary muscle
3 mitral valve
4 opening of coronary arteries
5 ascending aorta

Dissection of the right heart

A Sectioning and opening of the right auricle between the two venae cavae.

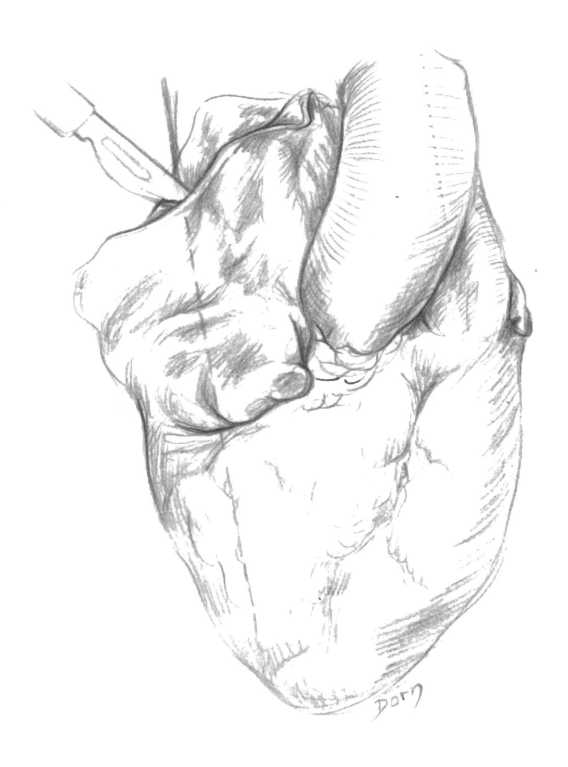

B The knife is introduced in the right auricle and the right ventricle is opened to the tip.

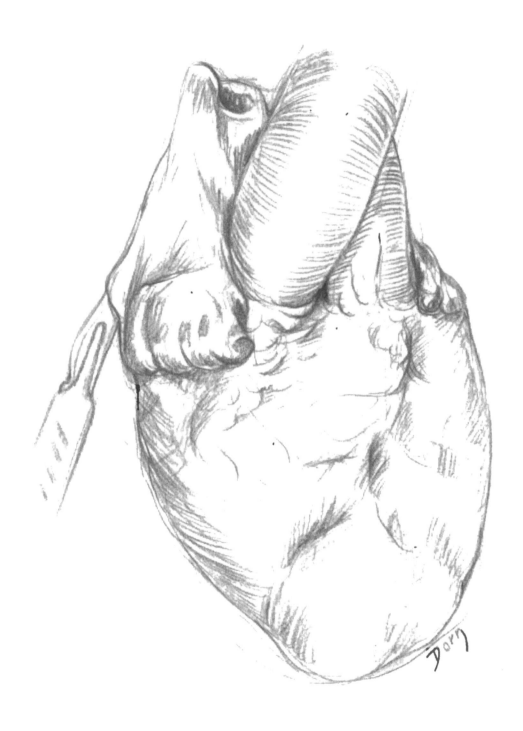

C, D The right ventricle is opened. The tricuspid valve and the papillary muscle are seen.

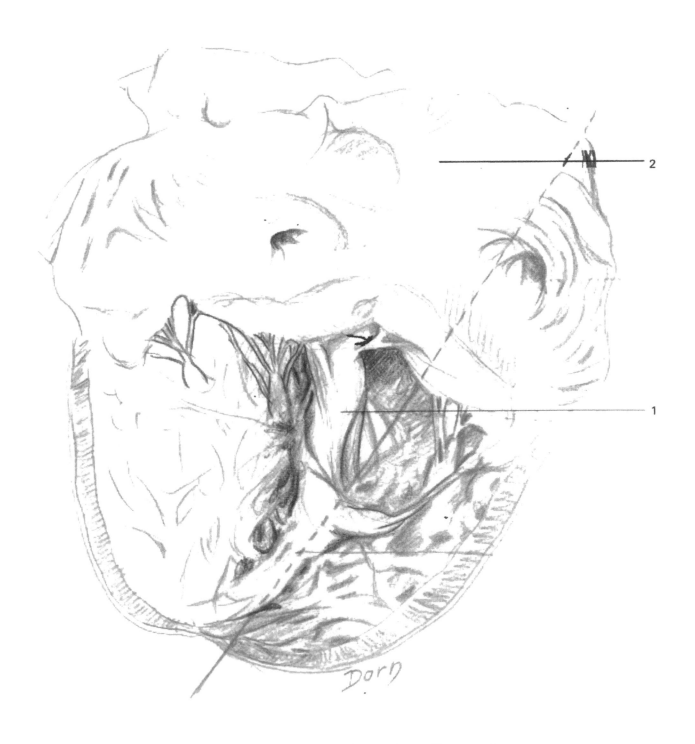

1 posterior papillary muscle
2 right atrium

D

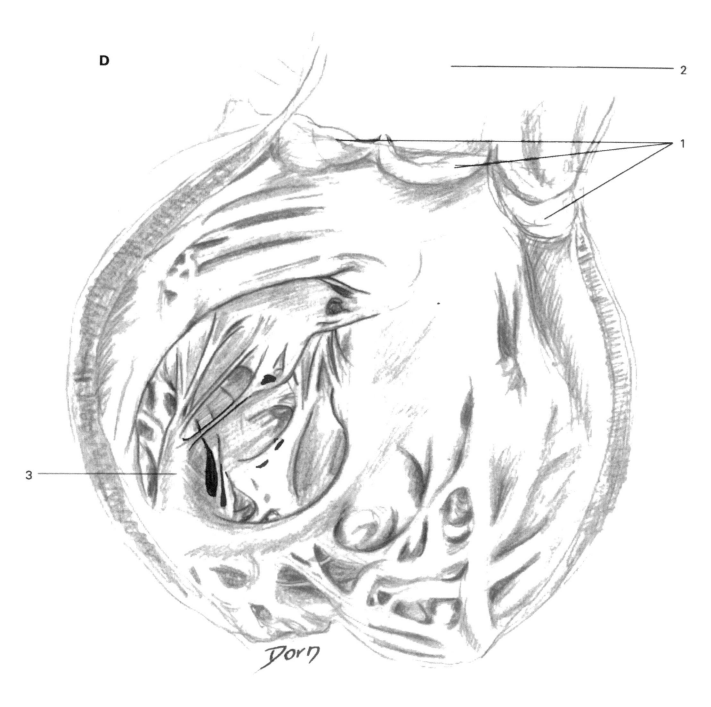

D

1 tricuspoid valve
2 right atrium
3 posterior papillary muscle

Index

Index

Index

Index

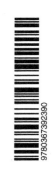